C PERFECT DAY

~

Knowing Nutrition Like The Back of Your Hand

Written by

Anthony E. Baucom

Edited by

Wenonah Garidel

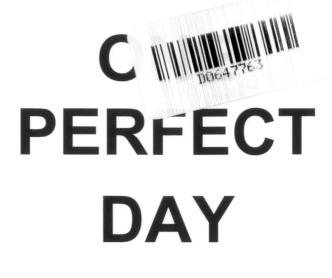
I0647763

Feed the mind. Free the body.

This book is dedicated to
the most lovely soul I have ever encountered,
my mother, Wenonah.

First Edition ©2012 by Anthony Baucom

Second Edition ©2013 by Anthony Baucom

Table of Contents

ONE PERFECT DAY

Knowing Nutrition Like The Back Of Your Hand

By Anthony E. Baucom

1. Introduction and "The Why"

Your health is a compilation of all the little decisions that are made in response to every situation that arises each day. Every one of those decisions impacts your total health. Essentially, they define you. In your hands, you have a book that contains a powerful, time tested and proven system for creating a tremendous and permanent change in the human body and mind. This change is obtained through educating yourself and holding yourself accountable for all the choices you make concerning your health. The awareness that you will gain from this simple process will give you the ability to naturally and "almost" automatically make the right decisions.

"One Perfect Day" is a system unrivaled in the world of health and fitness. Over the last twelve years and across the country, it has accrued well over ten thousand documented success stories that were facilitated by me personally. It is designed to empower you with the tools you need to match your commitment level, create results, and make the journey fun and easy. Without knowledge, commitment is unfocused, wasted energy, and knowledge is nothing without the wisdom for the application of that information to daily life. If I had readily accessible all the materials necessary to build a spaceship that could fly to the moon, I would fail in building it even if my commitment was at the highest level. My spaceship wouldn't even fly across the street because I have neither the knowledge nor the right plan. I would have to point my energy towards learning and probably working with someone who has already built and flown a spaceship or two successfully.

Some of your friends and family members might call you crazy for trying to achieve this goal and will actually try to hinder your progress just as if you really were trying to build a spaceship. It is imperative to keep the company and be in the environments that support you reaching your goals as often as possible.

In the field of the human body, I have flown more than ten thousand spaceships, and they have all arrived safely to their destinations. **You can trust this system**! I am an extremely reliable witness to its efficacy and safety. Your amazing body is far more complicated than building any spaceship, but this book boils down and simplifies all the information you need to understand and apply in order to create change that will last a lifetime.

After reading this book and applying the principles that are contained within, you will understand how your body works better than you ever thought possible and in a short amount of time. You will know more and have more ability than most when it comes to producing change and commanding performance of your incredible human body. As you progress, pin point your goal and set out on this journey and remember not to focus on the end result. Stay ever present and make sure you're following the guidelines closely and making the right decisions, right now!

THE WHY- Let me preface this by saying that this is not a diet. It is, however, a method of establishing aggressive accountability for your nutritional intake to create change, all the while becoming educated on not only *how* to create change, but *why* you should want to. The reasons why the program works so well is credited to the education and the system of accountability contained within, which in the beginning, are often disregarded and rejected. People sometimes say "can you just write down what I'm supposed to eat?" My answer is always a resounding "NO"! Understanding the rationale behind this system is a must to create results that last forever.

I have included only the information that you need to know in order to succeed. I promise that with just a little effort and patience, you will become completely self-sufficient for the rest of your life. So please, indulge me and know that I understand that you're in this for the results and not to become a nutritional scientist. This information will make the goals you achieve permanent, and the awareness gained will result in better automatic decision making skills. In fact, after achieving your goals and obtaining the education you need to sustain this new lifestyle, you can toss this book in the garbage. However, you will probably want to keep it because with all of its rips, tears and stains from being your constant companion, it will remind you of the incredible journey of discovery and change you have embarked upon.

This process of cultivating better nutritional habits will positively change many aspects of your life, and as a result of empowering your mind and body, you will see vast improvements in your family life, work life, and in your downtime.

Over the past twelve years, I have personally implemented this process (all over the U.S.) for well over ten thousand people who have come from all walks of life and have achieved a 100% success rate. **It never fails!** I cannot begin to describe the unbelievable changes I've witnessed in the lives of so many people as a result of this program's inception.

Prior to the publication of this book, my clients always told me "you have to write this all down," which is a phrase that they all hear from me on a regular basis regarding their food tracking. I learned from their input that the only thing this program was missing was a collection of information explaining all of the supporting information and the exact process I use to achieve these great results. They needed literature to reference that was easily accessible and could be found in one place, and so this book was born.

This book's compact size was designed specifically for the purpose of making it easy for you to carry it along wherever you go. In the back, there is a food journal that you will use to custom design and track your continuously evolving "perfect day" of nutritional intake using the information found within these pages.

"Everyone is different, what works for one person might not work for another." Right? Wrong! We are more the same than different. In fact, 99% of our genetic makeup is identical. Granted, genetically speaking, 1% can be a big deal but the emphasis that is placed on our differences regarding health and fitness is misguided, and this program proves that. Your focus should be placed on our similarities and not on that 1% because until you reach basic biochemical stability it means nothing. There exists a biochemical standard that must be achieved before even considering our differences. This 1% difference may be a factor for the performance athlete but the average person out there just wants to get back to optimal function, and so this book focuses on that larger population, but all of these same principles apply to athletes as well.

We are all human beings with the same physiological components, and we all live on the same planet to which we are connected. The very food you eat is made from the earth or should be if not processed beyond recognition. The earth has electric, colorful and action oriented days. It also has deep, dark nights for recovery from the day's activities and preparation for the action packed day to come. Remember that concept! It will mean a lot more as you learn the science behind how your body works. You will see the connection to the planet's cycles and your body's function.

The reason you're reading this book is to create change in your life and to generate movement in the direction of reaching your goals. Your goals may include anything from:

-       Reduction in body fat

-       Increasing   muscle   mass   and   athletic
performance

-       Managing your blood sugar, blood pressure or
cholesterol.

This will work for you.   Also, if you have a medical
condition, you are holding the perfect book, my friend!

In the case of special populations, the things you need to
do to cure certain health conditions are the same things
you should have done to prevent it.   You will easily be
walked down the path toward eliminating many of the
conditions that are plaguing this country such as: Type II
diabetes, obesity, high cholesterol and high blood
pressure just to name a few.   These are not diseases but
are conditions caused by a lack of knowledge and are
easily erased by knowing what you did to cause them in
the first place.   Whatever medical conditions you've
acquired over the years from lack of knowledge, this
book will fix quickly! There should be no deviation from
the proven and time-tested recommendations in this
book unless specified by your doctor.

There is a section on important considerations for
specific populations later in the book that will cover
information pertaining to high cholesterol, high blood
pressure and diabetes.   Many other conditions will be
eradicated as a byproduct of facilitating the needs of
your body that are being neglected right now. We all
have bad habits, some more than others, but a huge
percentage of the people that I work with have one or
more of those three conditions.   Just about all of them
believe these conditions are caused by genetic pre-
disposition.   They are wrong.   They all find out shortly
after symptoms begin to disappear, that blaming it on
genetics is just another lie we are told or tell ourselves.
There is however, some truth to genetic predisposition,
but there is far too much emphasis placed on it.   It's

more often used as an excuse for laziness and a lack of education than anything else. These conditions are stepping-stones to one another and are a result of the same bad decisions. When you become pro-active in using all of the many weapons that are available to you to fight the diagnosis, the condition(s) will either diminish greatly or vanish entirely. This system will give you these weapons! Just follow the simple steps, get immersed in the program and enjoy the unbelievable results.

As always, it is recommended that you consult your physician and get blood work done prior to beginning this program or any other (especially if there are special conditions involved) as well as set another appointment for sixty days out. That way, when you have your sixty-day checkup, you can thoroughly enjoy the astonished look on your doctor's face when he/she sees the incredible changes that have occurred in your overall health and appearance. At that time, you will also get to experience the joy of entirely or at least partially, removing the dependency you had on prescription drugs from your daily life. This will not be a temporary relief from your conditions as you've become accustomed to with the drugs. Drugs just sweep the symptoms under the rug but this program can eradicate them.

Ok. Let's get back on to the topic of good old fashion fat loss. Our mission right now is to get immediate results, create change, educate and motivate. We are not going for a 100% raw, seasonal, organic, locally grown, farm raised, and grass fed food just yet. But, I'll be honest; I hope to walk you as far into that direction as possible in the future. In the beginning, we must take baby steps.

The idea is that I meet you where you currently stand. Some people already have a lot of great habits and just need their lifestyle tweaked, while others are eating pizza for breakfast lunch and dinner or only eating one meal a day. You will learn how to design a perfect day of eating with foods you enjoy. As the results come, you will find yourself embracing the culture of living healthy and begin to migrate towards the healthier foods. After all, what's the more pressing issue, that you see results right away, or that you don't consume too much sugar, sodium or processed foods? You may think bars are a healthy substitute to processed snacks, but they can also be processed and are usually high in sugar and sodium. There are reasonable ones out there that are conveniently packaged for the fast paced life you live. However, in the future, you will see that preparation makes everything easier, and any kind of meal can be just as convenient and easily consumed as a bar if it is packed and prepared properly in advance. With a little extra preparation, we can avoid excessive amounts of packaged foods, which is always better. Now, I, along with you and your doctor will agree that seeing immediate results is what's most important. Striving for optimal intake is the truest respect you can demonstrate to the beautiful human body you have been given and we will move in that direction as you grow. All this will happen naturally as you progress. If your head is already there, that's great! If not, don't worry. We will get there. This will all be taken at your own pace.

2. Check your attitude! Push the reset button!

If you make a mistake and deviate from your perfect day, **do not be negative**…it's a complete waste of energy. Simply push the reset button and renew the commitment you made of progressing towards your goals. Too often people tend to beat themselves up over slip ups, or looking back at the mistake and getting frustrated. Look forward and do not waste your time and energy on being upset. Instead, harness and point that energy toward a productive end result. The only time you should feel a sense of really deviating from the path, is if you don't write down everything *including* your mistakes. Documenting your failures forces you to internally confront your actions and also allows for easier decision making when you confront the same issue in the future. Simply follow each easy step and stay positive. It is true that stress weakens our will power, but there are two kinds of stress, physical stress and perceived stress. Perceived stress is the kind of stress that hurts us the most. It is how you view stressors in your environment, but it's one you can control. You can't always change your environment, but you can change the way that you view it and manipulate the way it affects you. If you're in an environment that feels impossible to control, don't stress out. Assess each option available and in a relaxed fashion, rely on the skills you are about to acquire to determine the smartest choice. Trust yourself that you are doing the right thing based on the proven principles. Again, do not worry! This process is easy and fun if you keep your perceptions in check.

The Importance of exercise

Next up, in order of importance for overall health and wellness, is movement. This is not just about any kind of movement, but more specifically, the quality of movement. Education in this area is also fundamental. I'm currently working on a book that sums up all of the "must know" information regarding an exercise program design that creates positive forces on your body that counteract repetitive forces in your daily life. This method of resisted movements, combined with stretching techniques, creates balance and basically reverses the wear and tear on the body. The book will be called "The White Diamond Workout".

Until then, get active and stay active! Taking long walks and doing a mild full body resistance-training program three times a week is a great way to start. However, taking walks with postural awareness and resistance training paired with biomechanical knowledge is even better. Remember, this isn't just simply moving. Your goal should be about moving efficiently in order to maximize results. You should never just be "winging it" when it comes to your health and fitness. Get a good trainer who not only trains you but also educates you. Once again, you're looking for the "whys". Ask a ton of questions, look things up yourself when you don't understand and get into the culture. Don't be reactive about your health. Be proactive! I promise that you will be empowered by your efforts. However, don't get lost in the movement and allow your nutritional accountability and awareness to take the passenger seat. Nutrition is always number one! Thinking of exercise as a way to burn off your nutritional mistakes is a bad thought process to enter into and is the path to failure. Stay focused on your food input and your output will take care of itself. In fact, 70% of your caloric expenditure each day comes from keeping you alive. Movement is a much smaller piece of the "caloric expenditure pie" than people think. Support your metabolic requirements and the rest will all fall into place. Good nutrition will fuel movement and as your energy levels and athletic ability increase due to smart intake, you will *want* to move.

Let me reiterate, exercise is extremely important, but mechanical movement is nothing if not supported by chemical "fuel"...nutrients! Your results will come from your nutrition first, but exercise will help improve your quality of life and accelerate everything, as well as make the results last forever. Seventy percent of the calories you burn each day are to support your physiological functions and to keep you alive! If you feed that metabolic fire you will succeed. Exercise is of paramount importance, but at this moment, consciously put your focus on nutrition first and every one of your physical movements will matter more.

3. Establishing a Goal

How fast should you lose weight? What are healthy guidelines?

For women healthy range: **Body fat: 18-26%**

Over 50 years old up to 35%   **BMI: 20-25**

For men healthy range: **Body fat: 8-18%**

Over 50 years old up to 25%   **BMI: 20-25**

In order to establish an accurate goal, the first thing you need to do is get your base line statistics recorded. You need to know where you are before you really know where you're going. So, when you know exactly where you want to go, say it out loud and write it down. Consciously make an unwavering decision to achieve that goal. Then forget it! That's right, I want you to forget it and place **all** of your attention on the things that you need to do **today** to pull you closer to the end result. Do not focus on it but instead, focus on the next situation that will require a wise decision because if it hasn't already arrived, it is fast approaching.

Now, let's discuss how you will go about tracking the weekly physical statistics. You will need a scale, a bio electric impedance body fat analyzer and a measuring tape. Accurately obtaining measurements requires assistance and can be time consuming and inconsistent if done too often or by multiple people. So, the measuring tape will be used only once in the beginning to obtain a base line statistic and once after you have achieved your body fat and weight goals. You can buy an affordable BEI (bio electric impedance) tester online and if you use it on the same day of the week, under the same environmental conditions, it's a great tool for getting your starting statistics and monitoring progress. It also calculates your BMI (body mass index) for you. You can use a scale that has a body fat analyzer built in but make sure it's one of quality. Choose and use only one scale and body fat analyzer and be sure to keep all of your environmental influences consistent. Do not have your body fat tested with calipers or multiple BEI testers by random trainers at your gym because they will give you inconsistent readings due to varying skill sets and methods. We do not want anything affecting your motivation level while we push towards your initial adaptation. We need control, accountability and consistency. You will hear people shoot down the accuracy of BEI analyzers because they do have a margin of error of a couple of percent, but this is not important. The important thing is that you obtain and track your numbers using the same equipment, and always under the same conditions. At this point, perfect accuracy is not as important as is gathering the data in a controlled fashion and making sure that it is changing on a weekly basis.

When you are close to reaching or have reached your goals, then you can seek out other methods of assessing your body fat, such as calipers and hydrostatic weighing which, by the way, also have margins of error. To ensure optimal accuracy, there are certain things to keep in mind: environmental factors that should be consistent are time of day, sodium intake, water intake and level of activity. If one or more of these factor are inconsistent, it's not a big deal, just be aware of it and know that it can and will affect your body fat reading. The BMI will always be accurate because it's basically a math equation based on your height, weight and age. Your BMI and your scale weight are the numbers you need to watch, although, they can also be affected by water retention due to sodium intake and monthly cycle in women.

You will see a positive change weekly in all three numbers, but remember that your focus should always be on your monthly numbers and on the execution of your program because it's been proven to work time and time again. The three readings that should be tracked weekly are as follows:

1. Scale weight

2. Body fat

3. BMI

You will be losing weight at a rate of about 2.5 pounds a week if you are executing your program 100%, which is approximately ten pounds per month, give or take a pound. Sometimes the weight loss will be more dramatic in the beginning and then taper off to 10 a month, but you will not plateau if you're following directions. Even if you are following directions, never get discouraged by your weekly weigh in if it's not a full 2.5 lbs. Women can hold 1-3 lbs. of water when approaching and during menses and a little excess sodium can slip in and cause water retention as well. This will look bad on the scale, but means nothing in the grand scheme of things. It's the ten pound monthly goal that you need to make sure you're hitting. Watch your weekly changes too; they will be rewarding most of the time and therefore motivating.

Every little deviation from your perfect day will be a deduction from your results, remember that. Some of my clients get away with murder in the accountability department and still lose weight, but it will slow down if you don't stay sharp on tracking. Always keep in mind that you are and should be going after three goals: improving your overall health, performance and changing your body composition. Focusing on only one of these three is always to the detriment of the others, as is the case with almost all trendy, imbalanced diets and drugs/supplements.   We are looking for a positive, permanent adaptation in all of these areas, so be patient and do not look for ways to strip calories or try to find supplements that accelerate body composition change since this always leads to sacrificing health and performance.

4. Section One: Education and The Five Principles

What time did you get up this morning? Creating and maintaining biochemical stability.

1. Eating within a half an hour of waking- Lighting the fire!

It takes calories to breakdown food. That's right... the calorie is your friend if used properly. This breakdown is referred to as the thermic effect of feeding (TEF) and we are going to take full advantage of it by eating frequent and balanced meals starting with breakfast. Breakfast should be eaten within a half an hour of waking. One calorie is one unit of heat and the TEF basically works like this: In your cells you have Adenosine Di-phosphate (ADP) and free phosphates floating around in the cellular fluid (cytoplasm). As food enters your body, the hydrogen and carbon bonds, which are the backbone of the food's molecular structure, are broken. When this break happens, a little burst of energy is released which causes the ADP and a free phosphate to join together creating adenosine tri-phosphate (ATP) and ATP is essentially the energy currency in your body. The cell then breaks the ATP back down to ADP and a free phosphate and that break releases energy for function, and then the whole process starts over. It's an amazing process, right?

Think of your body like a shipping freighter. You need enough fuel for the motor to get you from Cheyenne, Wyoming to San Francisco, California, or in your body's case, you need enough blood sugar (glucose) to get you from 7am to 10am. No more fuel is needed when balanced correctly. After eating breakfast, we have lit our metabolic fire, and to maintain required levels of immediately available nutrients, you have to eat three hours later. So, when you get to 10am, it's time to refuel. Even though most of your calories used for daily activities come from stored fuel from the previous day, you need to maintain a balance of readily available, recently ingested carbohydrates (which breaks down to glucose) and protein (which breaks down to amino acids). Despite the fact that recently consumed foods make up a smaller piece of the pie as far as supporting immediate energy requirements (about 20%), if immediate resources in the blood fall too low, loss of lean mass, biochemical imbalance and metabolic burden will result.

The difference between your body and a shipping freighter is that if the freighter runs out of fuel it stops, but if your body runs out of fuel it begins to breakdown and consumes its own protein structures like muscle, to survive. Avoiding this state is of paramount importance, hence the frequent meals to maintain the stability of stored fuels and immediately available fuels. Your metabolism is a flame that burns like a candle at night. Within a half an hour of waking you need to turn that little flickering candle light into a blazing metabolic fire, or initiate your three hour glucose base. This fire can only be lit completely and for long durations by complex carbohydrates such as whole grain. Fat is burned in the fire of carbohydrates.

Our goal is to stimulate your metabolism. For your metabolism to be stimulated you must give it something to metabolize. When you rise in the morning and begin to move, those mechanical movements require chemical fuel (nutrients). If you light the fire earlier, you will burn more calories by the end of the day due to the TEF. All you have to do is make eating a balanced meal (containing complex carbohydrates) within a half hour of waking, a priority.

2. When active you must include complex carbohydrates (Whole grains are long chains) The fire starter!

Carbohydrates are gasoline for your metabolic motor or fire. All carbohydrates are sugar and all sugars are carbohydrates. There are very short chains of sugar that taste sweet so we call them "sugars" as they enter the blood stream fast and dissipate fast like a big fire that dies quickly. Then there are long chains of sugar that taste starchy and we call them carbohydrates. There are two kinds of long chain complex carbohydrates: fiber and starch. Fiber has no nutrient value for the body because it is in the form of cellulose (plant fiber) and cannot be broken down but, fiber has many other important functions which will be discussed later. Unrefined, complex carbohydrates (such as oats), breakdown and enter the blood stream slower due to containing fiber (cellulose) and having complex utilizable glucose which is slower to break down due to longer chains (starch).

These kinds of carbohydrates have a stabilizing effect on blood sugar due to their slower entry into the blood stream or time released effect (long burning fire). The complex carbohydrate is broken down first in the saliva. In fact, you could even say that the digestive process of carbohydrates begins prior to ingestion as the body begins saliva production in anticipation of sweet or starchy foods. As the long chains slowly break down, they are absorbed through intestinal walls into the blood stream which elevates blood sugar levels. The heart then pumps the glucose rich blood to all of the cells to nourish and support your body's energy requirements. Your brain and central nervous system rely solely on glucose, so as blood sugar levels increase to make glucose available to the cells, the pancreas releases insulin to meet the demand. Insulin is a hormone that like a "key", unlocks the cell walls where the glucose can then be utilized for energy.

17

The use of carbohydrates is to support activity which promotes the use of fat. By initiating and maintaining your glucose base throughout the day, you need complex carbohydrate to not only support basic activities but also to support brain and muscle function, and in the process, you will incinerate body fat. Fat is burned in the fire of carbohydrates. Essentially, as long as you keep breaking down and utilizing carbohydrates to support your movement, you are burning fat and protecting your lean mass from breakdown. Inversely, carbohydrate intake should drop dramatically when activity levels do. Once the sun goes down and you crash on the couch after work, carbohydrate intake should be reduced because, as discussed earlier, insulin is released to make glucose available to cells, but if you're not moving, your cells don't require it. Therefore, the insulin promotes the storage of that excess glucose in fat cells. Let's be honest, after dinner most of us do nothing but watch T.V. and go to bed, so why indulge in carbohydrates when your body does not require it? Less mechanical movement requires less gasoline… it's that simple. Carbohydrates are for action… they stimulate. Without action they are stored as fat.

As previously discussed, you are connected to this planet, and this planet has deep, dark nights that are necessary for the preparation and recovery from the explosive, active and colorful electric days. Wake up in the morning and stimulate (glucose) and when the sun goes down rehabilitate (protein). Avoid or lessen intake of invigorating foods and aromas because it'll set you up for a sound night's sleep and optimal recovery from the traumas of the day.

Your overall make-up transcends personality, spirit or anything else you believe. You are a compilation of cells and you need to feed your body with each cell in mind. If you took one muscle cell from your body and had to keep it alive for as long as possible, you would have to be sure that it had a steady supply of glucose or it would die. Your lean mass gives you the ability to function efficiently on this planet. It gives you the ability to combat all of the daily forces that influence you. Newton's laws are pushing you around all of the time, and your lean mass helps you to move efficiently in opposition to those forces. When it comes to fat loss and muscle gain, improving athletic performance, and avoiding or disposing of most conditions such as high blood pressure, Type II diabetes, etc... you must first manage your blood sugar.

3. Eating every 3 hrs. - Keeping the fire lit!

We have touched on the importance of initiating your glucose base (fire), but now we will discuss the importance of never letting that fire go out. Let's say you get up at 7:00 am and adhering to the program, you eat a meal that includes complex carbohydrates within a half hour of waking. So far, so good. As the whole grain slowly breaks down and trickles into the blood stream, the pancreas releases insulin to allow the entry of glucose into the cell which provides energy, protects lean mass and promotes fat usage. By 10:00 am, you are in danger of running out of your readily available blood sugar, so a re-initiating or stabilizing of your glucose base must happen. If not, the survival mechanism will soon be initiated and muscle mass will be catabolized (broken down). Organ and muscle mass, as well as connective tissue are broken down for fuel. If lean mass is repeatedly compromised in this way, over time, the reduction of lean mass results in decreased circulation, increased blood pressure, excessive body fat accumulation, and decreased muscular tension on the bone. This in turn results in a reduction of bone density and has an overall destructive impact on all of the body's functions. A reconstitution of your glucose base must happen at the three hour mark. Naturally, the time frame for entering a catabolic state varies depending on certain factors such as: genetics, digestive capabilities, quantity of calories consumed, macro-nutrient ratios of the meal, level of activity, etc. For example, an athlete usually eats even more frequently and in higher quantity to avoid becoming catabolic because of high activity levels. Entering a catabolic state promotes the storage of calories from the next meal, as a survival mechanism.

As if that wasn't bad enough, when the sun goes down, your body goes into a preparatory, repair mode to take stock of the day's traumas and deficits. The brain does not forget the fuel deficit that happened earlier in the day and begins to trigger cravings for sugar/carbohydrates at night to recover the body's glycogen. This occurs in case the same brain fuel catastrophe happens tomorrow, which is probable. The brain relies solely on glucose for function. What the brain sees is that it ran out of its primary fuel source and had to consume lean mass from the body and then had to store excess fat for survival. This lack of frequent intake and physiological support is common practice in our society and creates a "consistently inconsistent" environmental picture for the brain, so it begins to adapt. The more you store fat the less apt your body is to use it, especially when not exercising because exercise mobilizes stored fat for use.

This is a daily occurrence which happens multiple times a day and continues for years. The lean mass diminishes as the fat mass increases along with the life threatening conditions I've already spoken about. Managing your blood sugar is the first step to optimal physiological performance. Another extremely important factor related to frequent intake and blood sugar management is the production of pancreatic enzymes. In addition to producing insulin, the pancreas also produces enzymes that are extremely important in the digestive process. As time released carbohydrates break down, the pancreas works to produce small continuous outputs of insulin over long periods of time. This "motor like" action promotes the "churning out" of these highly valuable pancreatic enzymes. Going too many hours without eating allows the pancreas to "slack" in its insulin and enzyme production responsibilities which leaves you short on necessary enzymatic profiles. Deficiency in these important enzymes can lead to inefficient digestion, slowed metabolism and allergies. Therefore, eating every three hours and ensuring that your macro nutrient ratios reflect your activity levels is extremely important to implement into your lifestyle when beginning a march towards any improved physiological function. Whether it is fat loss, energy improvement, curing life threatening conditions, supporting and enhancing muscle mass and sports performance, it begins with blood sugar maintenance.

4. One fat source per meal, helping the fire burn longer!

Fat is an extremely important secondary fuel source to the carbohydrate. During long durations, lower intensity activities are "key" due to the fact that you burn larger amounts of fat than you do carbohydrates in that situation. However, even though fat is an energy superstar, in the absence of carbohydrates, the body burns fat less efficiently. Consequently, carbohydrates still hold the title of energy king. Fat slows the production of hydrochloric acid in the stomach which slows the whole digestive process to a simmer. This process helps to support the "timed release" of nutrients that enter the blood stream which is a wonderful benefit as far as blood sugar, amino acid pool stability, and pancreatic enzyme production and overall metabolic function is concerned.

Insulin can be toxic to cells in large quantities, whereas, fat and fiber can act as buffers to create an "arching effect" on the entry time into the blood stream on those high glycemic foods such as fruit juice or refined sugars/carbohydrates which can cause an unhealthy spike.

A great way to reduce acid reflux and G.E.R.D. is to make sure that a quality fat source is included with each meal. Another great benefit of having one fat source at every meal is to give you an easy way to manage the ratio of fat intake for the day between saturated fats and poly/mono unsaturated fats. Recommendations for total fat intake ratios are about 1/3 for each.

The cure for high cholesterol or bad LDL to HDL ratios in the blood is to ensure that you *overpower* the saturated fat with unsaturated fat. Mono unsaturated fats literally change low density lipoproteins (LDL) to high density lipoproteins (HDL) creating a "nonstick" environment for plaque in your arteries. Nothing that is whole is bad. In general, the only bad fats or foods are those that man has manipulated in some way. Saturated fat is known as bad fat but it also has many proven benefits such as assisting in stabilizing cell structures and lung surfactant which is an essential fatty fluid that lines the alveoli and bronchioles. In fact, your brain is largely made up of saturated fat. Of course, if excessive, it can kill you, but the same can be said for any fat, or any of the macro nutrients (carbs, fats, and protein), micro nutrients (vitamins and minerals) or just about anything in life for that matter.

The reason saturated fats have a bad rap is because it promotes an increase in LDL cholesterol which has been made dangerous by the traditional western diet of eggs, bacon and fried potatoes for breakfast, a bacon cheeseburger, fries and a shake for lunch, and steak with a "buttery" potato for dinner. This kind of intake contains poisonous amounts of saturated fat that will stop your heart. And, if you top that off with the refined carbohydrates in the shake, the white bread bun and the almost complete lack of fiber and color, you are in for serious health problems! Alone, saturated fat is not to blame but imbalance is the culprit and excess in any form always kills.

5. Having a plan based in proven science and maintaining total accountability!

Before you can create change you must have a plan based in proven science. Simply trying to track the caloric intake on your current path is not only a maddening full time job, but is the definition of insanity. To continue doing what you have been doing and expect a different outcome is crazy. All you will find out is what you already know...what you've been doing is not working. So let's begin rationalizing our game plan. Follow the simple criteria for the program design and always remember to make sure you understand why you are implementing each concept by referring back to the five principles. You **must** write down everything that passes through your lips even though it's the same food every day for a while. Your perception of reality when not logging is not reality. There are NO substitutions for two weeks after designing your first perfect day. Be sure that your level of hunger never exceeds a six or seven on a scale from one to ten on what I've dubbed your "hungometer". You should never go beyond a little hungry (6 or 7). Not only is it dangerous, but it will also slow your results for reasons I've already explained. Starving is unacceptable! It is detrimental to your physiological function and your success. You should arrive at each of your meals in anticipation. If you are not hungry, then you ate too much at the previous meal, and if you go beyond a seven on the "hungometer" before your next scheduled meal, then you didn't eat enough at the previous meal. This is how you will find your caloric requirement for the day. Learn to listen to your body and it will change your life.

5. Section Two: The Five Fingers

An easy way to remember how to prioritize your macro nutrient intake is by using your left hand as a reference. Your left palm up represents daytime and the back of your left hand signifies night. When the palm is up the **thumb** represents water. As water has no calories, it's not about caloric ratio, but rather a reminder that water is one of the five immensely important things you have to constantly focus on.

The **index finger** represents color (fruits and vegetables). Again, this finger is not so much about the ratio of calories but is a reminder of the eight mandatory servings that you **must** consume every day. The **middle** and longest finger symbolizes complex carbohydrates. This is where the loose caloric ratio for meals kicks in. Carbohydrates are the longest finger and a priority during the day/activity because that is when your body uses them most efficiently. You must keep your immediately available blood glucose levels stable. Remember, fat is burned in the fire of carbohydrates.

The **ring finger** represents fat. The length of the ring finger compared to the length of the middle finger is a general guideline for the calories needed from fat in a daytime meal compared to the calories from carbohydrate. Finally, the **pinky** is protein, but this is not to say that protein is not important in the day. As we know from previous reading, amino acids are always being depleted and need to be maintained through constant protein intake. This is in no way exact, but it is a great mental picture that will help to keep your priorities in order.

At night the hand flips over. Protein takes priority as the middle finger. Fat stays the same as the ring finger and color as the index finger. Carbohydrates become the pinky. This does not mean that you can't have a small controlled amount of carbohydrate at dinner, but

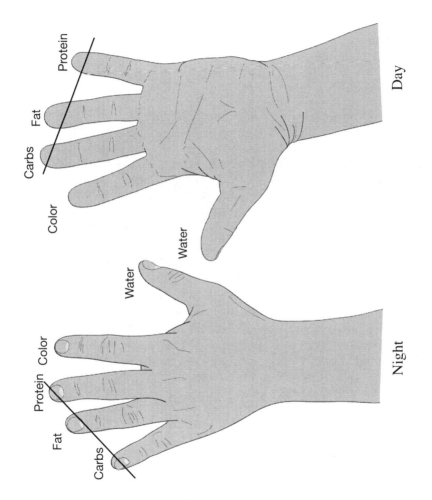

25

remember that your body doesn't use them efficiently when you're not active, and instead of the insulin response assisting the cells (using the glucose) it will promote its storage in fat cells. So minimize them at dinner; in fact, I often cut grains and potatoes out completely at dinner and rely solely on the carbohydrates (fiber and sugars) in vegetables. You can use this quick reference model to close each finger one by one like a check list until you've made a fist and trust that you have designed a balanced meal, anywhere, anytime.

1. The Thumb: Water

With the body being about 75% water, water is the basis for all bodily fluids and is the regulator of all of the body's function. Water is essential for the body to support energy transport and toxin removal for every cell in the body and the conducting of electrical currents that facilitate life. Water also dilutes toxins such as ureic acid and allows for easier processing for the kidneys and liver. It's important to be aware that every single chemical process in the body is facilitated by vitamins interacting with enzymes. They rely on water to get them to their proper places in proper time. Think of all the cells in your body as the buildings in the city of Venice. Enzymes are the mayor and the vitamins are the guy driving the gondola. The intercellular fluid is the canals, and if the canals are dry the mayor has a hard time getting around taking care of the city's business. The import of goods (nutrients) and the exports of waste… well, you get the idea. It is very important! Shoot for 96oz. If you fall short or go over a little, it's no big deal but still make it a serious focus. If you find yourself running to the bathroom more than you used to, you have improved your intake. Recommendations for water intake vary depending on a number of factors but this seems to be a good number to achieve for just about anybody. I'm almost 6' 4"and require every bit of that 96oz, but I fall very short regularly and have to constantly remind myself to keep water close.

2. The Index Finger: Color (fruits and vegetables, enzymes, vitamins, minerals and phytonutrients)

Don't get too stuck on green! Each and every different color of fruits and vegetables is indicative of a different enzymatic, vitamin, mineral and phytochemical profile. Each color is a different signature blend of earth chemicals specially designed to nourish your body's needs. As a species, our last bastion of hope is to hold on to our only remaining connection to the earth from which we come. Delicious and beautiful looking fruits and vegetables are full of phytonutrients, poly-phenols called bioflavonoids. Bioflavonoids have a host of incredible health benefits due to their antioxidant, anti-inflammatory, anti-bacterial, antiviral, and anti-allergenic properties. They have been proven to fight cardiovascular disease, cancer and osteoporosis to name a few. The old recommendation of five daily servings of fruits and vegetables is dead and gone, as are the days of good nutrient density of our fruits and vegetables that our grandparents were accustomed to.

It is estimated that an apple today has about ten percent of the nutrients that an apple had one hundred years ago as a result of over worked land, genetic modification, pesticides, hydroponics and manures. Subsequently, the recommendation is now eight to ten servings and only three from fruit because of the impact of the sugars on the body. The rule with sugar is that they have to come with a benefits package of fiber and nutrients. However, as technology gets more involved and the year's progress, the negatives of the high sugar content are beginning to outweigh the benefits of the nutritional benefit.

Fruit is by no means, bad for you. In fact, it is great for you. But consume fruit mainly in the daytime or early evening so that the sugar gets utilized through activity and insulin levels stay down when inactive, thus avoiding fat storage. Large amounts of fructose intake results in the conversion of some triglycerides (the body's storage of fat). Always eat the whole fruit, don't drink just juice, this way you accompany the sugars with fiber. You generally shouldn't be drinking your calories anyway. To sum up colors... eat colorfully! You need a broad spectrum of vitamins, minerals and phytonutrients and that's a sure way to get them.

Eat fruits and veggies that are in season as much as possible. Out of season fruits and veggies require manipulation to grow using fake light environments and chemicals. They can be imported with chemicals on them that aren't even legal for use in the U.S. Eat organic if you can. Organic has no chemicals, more nutrients and flavor, but can be costly. If you must choose, buy organic dairy and meats because the inorganic dairy and meats typically have 20 times more pesticides than organic fruits and veggies. Finally, be sure to pair fruits with a fat and protein and remember how fruits and vegetables are built. They contain complex carbohydrate but it is in the form of fiber and the rest of the carb content is short chain sugar. Obviously, there is more sugar in fruit than veggies, so they do not qualify as a source to support your blood sugar for long durations. There is no substitute for complex carbohydrates that are rich in fiber and starch for that job, such as whole grains.

3. The Middle Finger: Carbohydrates (breaks down to glucose and stored as glycogen)

In order to have optimal fat burn, the presence of carbohydrate is necessary. The brain and other tissues of the central nervous system cannot store glucose locally but are almost solely dependent on it for function. Therefore, a constant supply is a must. Even though the fuel required for a majority of daily activity comes from stored fuel, a constant maintenance of blood sugar is mandatory to support immediate energy requirements, brain function, and metabolic activity. In fact, your brain and red blood cells rely on the glucose from your last meal.

Another very important factor to remember is that an inadequate amount of carbohydrate intake can cause the lean mass (muscle, organs and connective tissue) to atrophy, which can, in turn, negatively affect every physiological function of the body. On top of that, if you experience a decline in blood sugar during the day, big time cravings can result later on in the evening. This is the why you get those insatiable cravings for anything carbohydrate/sugar flooding in when you get home after work and are defenseless against them. It's not because you are weak and have poor will power. It's not because you are an emotional eater. You are simply a victim of the bad decisions that you made earlier in the day when you decided not to eat within a half an hour of waking or when you decided to skip that snack and go six long hours without reconstituting your glucose base. It's also the bad decision of not including any whole grain with that chicken salad you had for lunch. But now you know. Now you are educated and can put a stop to those negative patterns with your newfound awareness. Now you know that if you don't support your day, you will lack control at night as your brain tries desperately to recover its glycogen, the storage form of glucose. You then pay dearly for a pattern of decisions that have dire consequences. This pattern is responsible for most of the medical conditions that that are now in epidemic proportion. Are you going to get up tomorrow and not eat? I think not.

As previously discussed, all carbohydrates are sugar and all sugars are carbohydrates, and it all breaks down to glucose. The important thing to remember is that unrefined complex carbohydrates (organic if possible) such as brown rice, whole wheat, oats and quinoa are your focus due to their slow, time released entry into the blood stream. The entry of complex carbohydrate into the blood is slower due to the fiber content and the complex long chain molecular arrangement. The fiber content can also bind with some of the ingested fats of a meal, carrying them out of the body before being absorbed.

Another huge benefit that comes along with unrefined carbohydrates is the high amount of vitamins and minerals that facilitate enzymatic function which makes us more metabolically active. This is yet another example of how carbohydrates stimulate the metabolism. Complex carbohydrates increase satiety, stabilize blood sugar, improve body composition and have a high thermic effect of feeding. However, in times of inactivity, carbohydrates and insulin is a recipe for excessive bodily fat gain and health problems. A balanced intake to support your activity levels is the key. As the body likes to keep glucose levels in the blood stable (about 20g), a limited daily intake of 130g per day has been issued and recommended by the American Dietetic Association. This recommendation would change, of course, depending on individual goals and requirements. Maintaining blood sugar levels is one of the most beneficial and highest physiological priorities.

Fiber: The real story

There are two types of fiber: soluble and insoluble. Soluble fiber has the ability to lower cholesterol and keep your arteries clean. Insoluble fiber is a complex carbohydrate that cannot be broken down by your body because it's in the form of cellulose (plant fiber), kind of like paper. Only three percent of insoluble fiber will be converted into utilizable glucose; therefore, it has next to no nutritional benefit. Increasing your fiber intake is important, but it should be gradual and accompanied by increased water intake to avoid bloating. The bacterial effort in the intestines to breakdown insoluble fiber is a good thing. It creates gasses and promotes intestinal motility which cleanses the colon. It also works by entangling water and food particles in a "net" as they pass through the intestines creating a "timed release" effect on absorption of nutrients into the blood stream. This has a stabilizing effect on blood sugar and insulin levels and we know from previous reading just how important that is. Fat tends to bind to insoluble fiber as well and is carried out of the body as waste before being absorbed.

Both forms of fiber are of incredible physiological importance but have no direct nutrient value. In fact, over use of fiber to feel "full" is a bad way to think despite the media and various food manufacturers bombarding us with false information on a regular basis. More fiber is not always a good thing. Eating more whole foods that are high in fiber is a fantastic idea because when the fiber is accompanied by a significant source of utilizable carbohydrate and micronutrients (vitamins and minerals), and nutrient density, that is what will support your physiological requirements.

On the other hand, eating packaged, processed, fiber enhanced foods can be a detriment to your health if taken out of balance. Beware of low carbohydrate breads, tortillas, cereals and pastas because all they're doing is using a type of paper as filler, and robbing you of the nutrients that your body needs, not to mention, your hard earned cash. When reading labels, fiber and sugar need to be subtracted from the total carbohydrate to get the amount of glucose sustaining carbohydrate. One whole wheat tortilla that has 10g total carbohydrate, 8g of fiber and 1g of sugar, leaves you with only 1g of actual whole wheat. This is completely imbalanced because wheat does contain fiber in its proper ratio with starch (when in its natural state) but, by adding too much fiber nutrient, density is reduced. So, yes, it's high in fiber and low in sugar but where are the vitamin and mineral profiles and glucose support that your brain and muscles require to function? Low sugar and high fiber is a good thing when in proper balance with utilizable complex carbohydrate. Be an aware shopper and label reader.

4. The Ring Finger: Fats/Lipids (breaks down to fatty acids- stored as triglycerides)

The ratio of intake of mono unsaturated fat, poly unsaturated fat and saturated fat is extremely important. Out of all of the fat consumed in your day, you should be striving for around a third to come out of each day. Quality fats contain EFA's (essential fatty acids) and serve a vast amount of physiological purposes. Omega-3 and Omega-6 oils are the two main types of EFA's. Once in the body, they are converted to prostaglandins that regulate inflammatory states and tons of metabolic functions. Omega-3 fats are naturally ant-inflammatory, whereas, some omega-6 fats are said to be pro-inflammatory. Therefore, balancing these fats is also important. If you are keeping cellular inflammation in check it means there will be more efficient physiological function. Saturated fats are usually solid at room temperature, whereas, unsaturated fats are usually liquid.

The synthetic process of hydrogenating unsaturated fats by adding hydrogen molecules is done to keep them solid at room temperature, (like margarines) and to help prevent them from becoming rancid. This process changes the shape of the organic oil molecule which becomes hard for our bodies to breakdown and negatively affects function. These odd shaped molecules can become foreign bodies. Processed, manipulated fat is the only bad fat. Any food product is healthier when it is more whole and less touched by man's processed fingers.

Fats slow the production of acids in the stomach which causes a sluggish breakdown and absorption of glucose into the blood, thus creating a stabilizing effect on blood sugar levels. This action on the acid levels of the stomach can also help to inhibit acid reflux when fat is distributed in even amounts throughout the day. Fat has many other benefits other than simply being delicious. It is a great source of energy, insulates the body against heat loss, helps absorb fat soluble vitamins A, D, E, and K, and provides you with a feeling of satiety. Saturated fat is good for you too. Intake of saturated fats have been shown to protect the liver from alcohol, prescription drugs and other toxins, as well as cause liver cells to eject fat content, and helps with fatty liver and stimulates immune function and metabolism. Saturated fat also makes up a large percentage of cell structures and in the right amounts has a stabilizing effect on cholesterol levels and sex hormones. It also provides 100% of the coating necessary in the lungs airspaces called lung surfactant. Without proper amounts of lung surfactant or a surfactant made up of the wrong fatty acids, the lungs cannot function properly and this can lead to many health problems such as asthma. Saturated fat is also tasty and a great source of energy. It can be used to fry foods (olive oil) at a much higher heat than unsaturated fats without breaking down.

Unsaturated fats have a low heat threshold and breakdown easily causing cross bonding of molecules when cooled, thus making it hard for the body to process. Saturated fats have been demonized for their role in elevating LDL or bad cholesterol. However, they are very important for maintaining the bio-chemical balance we should all be striving for. And by the way, your brain is largely made up of saturated fat! As you can see, these fats aren't taboo... they simply need to be balanced. Egg yolk, dairy, beef, dark meat chicken, and heavy cream are delicious and nutritious, and they also contain unsaturated fats. Unsaturated fats are indeed as magical as you have heard, but were until recently, looked down upon as badly as saturated fat is now. Due to their tendency to breakdown fast in high heat and become rancid, these fats are healthiest when raw or cooked at very low heat. That's why saturated fat is used to fry food. It can be used many times at high heat before breaking down.

Mono-unsaturated fat and poly unsaturated fats are liquid at room temperature and semi-solid when cooled. Some excellent sources include avocado, salmon, seeds, nuts, olive oil, canola oil, sunflower oil, and surprisingly, beef fat and lard! Many saturated fat sources also contain substantial amounts of unsaturated fat. Important for its ability to lower LDL cholesterol and raise HDL cholesterol, unsaturated fats also have many other incredible benefits including natural anti-inflammatory properties, absorption of calcium and fat soluble vitamins, cardiovascular benefits, and much more.

5. The Pinky Finger: Protein (breaks down to amino acids- amino acid pools)

Protein breaks down to amino acids which build and repair damaged tissues, and in fuel shortage situations, it can even provide energy. Your muscles and organs are all comprised of proteins which are created from and maintained by amino acids. The amino acids talent doesn't stop there. Everything from chemicals in the body (such as hormones and enzymes) to structures of the body is made up of proteins. As protein breaks down into amino acids and enter general circulation, they are added to amino acid pools in blood plasma. These pools of amino acids must be constantly maintained through protein intake. Our bodies need to maintain about 100g of amino acids in the blood plasma pools so that they can be exchanged from the blood into the cells of tissues and then back into the blood for the production and distribution of enzymes, hormones, antibodies, structural proteins (muscle), organs and connective tissues. If protein intake and consequently, amino acid pools fall too low, the body begins to breakdown muscle, organ, and connective tissue in order to fill the requirements amino acids need to function. This is but another central reason to eat every three hours.

Out of the 20 amino acids needed, 12 of them can be made by your body, but the other 8 needs to be acquired through daily food intake. For this reason these 8 are known as the *essential* and the other 12 as the *nonessential*. Foods that contain all 8 essential amino acids are said to be complete, fish and chicken are good examples, and intake of complete proteins (many from animal sources) are an easy way to meet requirements. However, there are many foods from plant sources that contain quality amino acid profiles, and when paired with each other (like beans and rice) they can become complete and satisfy amino acid pool requirements.

However, the jury is still out on whether or not these food pairs need to be eaten at the same time or throughout the day to be optimally effective. The latest and strongest evidence that I have seen suggests that eating them together best supports amino acid pool requirements. Just like when carbohydrate levels fall too low, if protein levels fall too low we begin to cannibalize ourselves. As lean mass is sacrificed, our experience on this planet is sacrificed because it is our lean mass which gives us the ability to effortlessly oppose and overcome all of the forces that are pushed upon our bodies every moment of every day.

Contrary to current trends, the body does not require the excessive amounts of protein for function or development. However, it is of the utmost importance to maintain the amino acid pool in the blood. While fats can be easily stored in large quantities and carbohydrates in small quantities, protein cannot be. A minimum daily protein recommendation of 0.8 grams per kilogram of body weight, or 55 grams for a 150lb individual has been issued for amino acid pool maintenance. Requirements increase as activity levels increase as do the needs of carbohydrate and fat. As always, our mantra is about keeping balance. There is a lot of discrepancy in the scientific world regarding high protein intake. For example, historically, people trying to gain muscle mass have relied on the 1g per pound of body weight method which takes our 55g for our 150 pound person to 150 grams. This type of top heavy protein intake has been frowned upon in recent years for the reasons that high protein intake can dehydrate and rob your bones of calcium, hurt your kidneys and cause a myriad of other health issues. However, there is some recent research that opposes these allegations in the healthy body that leads us to the problem.

All of these studies are subjective and rely on data that is contingent on too many factors. For example, a high protein diet can be hurtful to an elderly individual who has kidney, immune system or bone density issues, but helpful to an elite athlete whose focus is performance. The problem is that most of us fall smack in the middle. Perhaps we have too much fat on our bodies resulting in high cholesterol and/or blood pressure, and yet we are at the gym making attempts at athletic activity. No matter where you fall in the scope of things, whether you're leaning more towards the athlete, more toward the sedentary or an "issue laden" individual, the solution is balance. Everyone can benefit from improved balance in lifestyle decisions. Protein, fat and carbohydrates complement each other and we are going to discover how to balance these nutrients in the way that best compliments your level of activity. We will accomplish this using a simple method that will cause all of this to simply fall into place.

In summary:

Within a half an hour of waking, your metabolic fire *must* be lit. Take it from a flickering light to a raging, blazing, brain function supporting, energy requirement fulfilling and blood sugar stabilizing fire! Only carbohydrates can light that fire. As you breakdown the complex carbohydrate, glucose slowly trickles into the blood stream, the heart pumps the nutrient rich blood around your body, the pancreas releases insulin that will open the mouths of the cells which allows them to utilize the fuel. Fat is burned in the fire of carbohydrates. Now that you have your furnace lit, you need to keep it lit. You need to re-initiate your glucose base and amino acid pools every three hours or else pay dearly by losing lean mass that you should be protecting and ensuring that your quality of life is high in the midst of ever present forces. Make sure carbohydrates are consumed during the day (activity) and that intake of carbohydrate is reduced at night (inactivity). Get one fat source per meal but *only* one. There should be no fat free meals. This will help to keep your calorie intake controlled and make it easy to keep track of the ratio of fats consumed and ensure you're getting all of the fantastic benefits. Protein at every meal is an absolute must as well, and as activity and calories from carbohydrate intake decreases, calories from fat and protein will take their place. It just makes sense when you think about it, and it has been a pleasure to see this simple information create such tremendous change in so many lives. But before you even start to apply what you're learning, you must have a concrete plan complete with goals and timelines *for* those goals. It's time to learn exactly how, now that you know the why. It is now time for program design and preparation guidelines. This is when your plan will start to take shape.

6. Section Three: Program Design Introduction

It is time to get into program design, so let's get the ball rolling! Some of you are probably saying "It's about time!" Right? And now you're laughing because I busted you on it. It was all important information, trust me, and it will act as a great reference if you ever forget why you're doing things the way you are or have to explain to others why you're doing what you're doing. In order to gain accountability you must first lose variety. When you begin to get a handle on the concepts and see and feel the results of your efforts, variety will come.

For the sake of controlling your environment you have to start out simple. Make no mistake about it though… you cannot eat the same foods for the rest of your life. Your body requires a broad spectrum of nutrient sources. We will begin to cycle new foods in as soon as you become more comfortable with your initial perfect day. However, for at least the first couple weeks of this program, you will eat the same thing every day.

We will create a perfect day and execute it. Your first goal is creating your perfect day. Your second goal is one perfect day of nutritional intake and the tracking of every single unit of heat (calorie) that passes your lips. Your third goal will be one perfect week of intake and tracking. Touch nothing other than the meals you decide upon for that week and maintain absolute accountability for every calorie. It doesn't matter what other people are doing because you are on a mission. You have goals and are committed to them! It is not pleasure time for you. Instead, it is time to follow the five simple principals to perfection because they will take you to what you want and need.

Nothing tastes better than how you are going to feel. You can stick to those same foods beyond the first week if you want. In fact, a lot of people find that once they

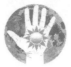

have meal choices that are working for them they like to stick to them, but you cannot repeat the same perfect day of eating for more than four weeks. After that initial time, you will need to start putting together new meal options and implementing them. Remember that it's not the particular foods that are getting you the results. It's the way you are pairing your macronutrients to support your lifestyle...your "fuel mixture". There are millions of food combinations that will create the same great results and they are just as easy to eat when you're busy as long as you have prepared them. A yogurt, granola and berry meal is no simpler to whip out and eat the following day than a Thanksgiving dinner if you've packed and prepared it the night before. These changes in your plan must happen to ensure that your body is getting the broad spectrum of nutrients from the different required sources. Also, eating the same foods every day and for too long, can promote the development of allergies.

7. 1200 to infinity: No caloric limit

How many calories should you be eating per day and per meal?

We are going to let your body decide how much it needs by improving your communication with it. Eating processed foods coupled with bad timing, eating imbalanced meals, intake of fake sweeteners and many other factors throw off body chemistry and can adversely affect your ability to communicate with your body. We are going to fix that and sync you up to your body's needs because believe me, it will tell you if you listen. First we have to re-establish the connection. Everyone's activity level varies, not only person to person, but day to day. There is no metabolic calculation or recommended amount of grams of nutrients that can take all of your personal environmental data into account. Therefore, we will make sensible decisions while designing your initial perfect day and learn to really listen to your body so we can tweak your program to fit you.

First of all, there really are no such things as snacks. They are all meals and a good, safe starting point is between 250 and 300 calories per meal. About 1,200 - 1,500 calories per day is a good starting point for most people. However, as you learn to use your "hungometer" (next section) to manipulate your meals by listening to your body, you may find that you go slightly below the 1,200 calorie mark and still feel great. Do not be alarmed! 1,200 calories is not all you're eating, it's all you're ingesting. We are going to make sure that our food choices are nutrient dense and let the other necessary calories come from your body fat. You will be devouring the contents of your fat cells and one pound of fat is roughly 3,500 calories. If you go a little above the 1,500 calorie mark, don't sweat it! You're getting adjusted and can adjust your aggressiveness as time progresses. Bottom line is you will succeed. When the fat falls off the beautiful muscle, it will remain due to the protection provided by your protein intake, blood sugar management and your ability to listen to your body.

It is important to remember that the 1,200 calorie bottom is there for a reason. Our metabolisms respond to intake. Getting too aggressive and ingesting far too few calories to support basic requirements causes cannibalization of body structures, but it also causes reduced thyroid hormone output. This reduced benefit of the thermic effect of feeding is essentially a slowing of the metabolism, which is the opposite of what we are looking for. Increasing your calories has the opposite effect and is sometimes exactly what is needed to stimulate your metabolism and accelerate fat loss! Do not be afraid of calories. They are simply tools at your disposal that will sustain your body's needs, help you achieve your goals, and be delicious while they do it.

8. THE "HUNGOMETER"

Listening to Your Body: "On a scale of 1-10"

A great way to start really communicating with your body is to ask yourself how hungry you are on a scale of 1-10. You should never go past a six or seven on your "hungometer". Trust the first number that pops into your head when asking yourself this question. If that number is close to seven, you need to eat. Break the "three hour rule" if it's necessary to manage your blood sugar and amino acid levels. It's always ok to eat early but never ok to eat late. However, if you're below six, and can wait until your designated mealtime, do so. Going past seven indicates you have a near empty gas tank and are hurting progress. Your body is letting you know that will soon be compromising the lean mass we are trying to protect. It is a very dangerous place to be, especially when active, but active means *drastically* different things for different people.

Being in the fitness industry, I have called the ambulance countless times for people who black out in the gym and hit the floor after going too long without fuel. Even if you're not working out it makes you vulnerable. If you eat your breakfast at 6 am and by 8:30 you are approaching a seven you must eat early. Tomorrow you will add a little more carbohydrate or protein to your breakfast, and if the same thing happens at night increase protein but keep carbohydrate intake low. If the opposite occurs, and after eating breakfast you're a two on the "hungometer" and you're not anticipating your next meal at the three hour mark, you ate too much for breakfast. Still eat your meal, and the next day back off the calories in your breakfast so that you arrive at your next meal-time mildly hungry, and simply anticipating the meal. Use your "hungometer" to manipulate your program to fit your lifestyle and trust what your body has to say.

9. IT'S TIME FOR PROGRAM DESIGN!

The first page of your food log lets you design your first perfect day to act as a constant reminder and first model of what perfect is. Each step will include notes that will help you along. Follow the process to perfection, no side steps! You can use the sample perfect days and simply adjust them to your liking or come up with your own creations using the criteria. The sample days are examples of the kind of meal choices and perfect days that thousands of people have chosen to start with and they all achieved their goals, quickly and safely. All meals are interchangeable from sample day to sample day as long as you exchange lunch for lunch, dinner for dinner etc. keeping the macro nutrient ratios consistent and the five principles intact. After a while, you will be able to create your own balanced meal plans with ease. Let's get started!

Step 1: Choose something easy to prepare within a half hour of waking and make sure that whole grain is included along with a fat source, protein source and a "color" such as:

- 1/2 cup of cooked oats

- A tablespoon of peanut butter or almond butter

- ½ cup of blue berries or ½ of a banana

You can even add a ½ cup of fat free milk or a little chocolate protein powder to the meal for a little extra protein, in addition to the protein content in the peanut butter. Write it down on page one, square one, and list each item separately with caloric values next to each. It will be your only breakfast choice for one-two weeks, so make sure that you enjoy your meal choices. Don't choose foods because you think they are the healthiest thing in the world but rather stick to what you know and love that meets the criteria. You need to enjoy each meal. For example, if you don't like oatmeal, don't eat it! Instead choose a grain that you enjoy then add the protein, fat source and color because the first 21 to 30 days are *so* crucial to create this adaptation!   We are going to make this painless, easy and enjoyable!

Be sure to remember the left hand macro-nutrient ratio recommendation for your level of activity/ time of day. You must get carbohydrates, color, fat, and protein in proper amounts. Other examples could be:

1)   1 cup cereal, ½ cup 1% milk, and 1/3 cup blue berries

2)   1 whole wheat wrap, 3 egg whites, ½ oz. cheese (one ounce is the size of a matchbox), and ¼ cup peppers and onions

3)   1 slice whole wheat toast, 1 tablespoon peanut butter and ½ of a green tipped banana.

Even though these combinations have varying values of fat and protein, the quality carbohydrates are dominating the ratio like protein does as the day progresses. Just make sure that your fat and protein sources are present and substantial. You can enhance proteins at breakfast using egg whites, protein powder, fat free milk etc. When personally designing plans, I often don't enhance the breakfast with more protein until after things are further along just to avoid the extra step. Right now, it's all about protein intake and keeping things simple because it will always get a lot heavier later in the day anyway.

Important Preparation Notes: Make a big batch of oatmeal on Sunday for the week if time doesn't permit it in the morning. Chop the peppers and onions the night before, be prepared. Leave a measuring cup on your kitchen counter. It will help with easy and exact meal preparation and teach you how to eyeball portions over time. Remember that this is a great time to include fruit for its metabolism stimulating qualities! **Note:** Green tipped bananas have longer chain sugars than brown spotted ones.

Step 2: Decide on the snack that you will be eating three hours after breakfast. The same ratio rules apply. Make it something easy to throw in a bag the night before. For example:

a) ¾ cup low fat cottage cheese with 1/3 cup fruit or veggie and whole grain crackers

b) ¾ cup of 2% Greek yogurt with 1/3 cup of low fat cereal and ¼ cup blue berries.

If the yogurt is 0% fat then you can use granola for your fat and carbohydrate but be wary of the sugar! If it's a flavored yogurt, you would use maybe a tablespoon of shaved almonds or a teaspoon of flax seed for the fat (no sugar) and a low sugar cereal. You can't put a sugary granola on top of a sugary yogurt with berries which also contain sugar. Something as simple as a bar (not high in sugar) which is nutritionally balanced, easily packed and meets the basic criteria can be a viable choice for meal number two if the bar contains whole grain. **Note:** I sometimes allow for a little extra sugar at first for ease of packing and to make sure that the individual actually enjoys their day of eating and will adhere to the program. Let's face it, what's more important, avoiding a little extra sugar or creating results and obtaining an education that will change the trajectory of a life? I always walk my clients towards an organic, low sugar way of thinking because as the results begin to flood in, they develop a respect for the value of truly taking care of their bodies, and the joy of that feeling empowers them to stay the course. Soon, you will see that you can make a million different things out of any meal. Sometimes I will pack a little left over dinner from the previous night and just add a little bit of carbohydrate like sweet potato, quinoa, brown rice etc. With just a little added effort, I can make an even more nutritious and delicious meal, and it only takes 5 minutes to pop open and eat. **Note:** Watch out for bars that are too low in calories. Remember, it's a meal and it needs to meet that criterion.

Step 3: Choose a lunch. Keep in mind that carbohydrates are nonetheless important because you still have plenty of active day left. It's important not to get caught up on using the examples provided. Of course, you can use them for the first couple of weeks up to a month, but then you need to branch out into different foods and learn to apply the concepts you have learned toward them. The sky is the limit when it comes to lunch because it's for *all* five of your meals. I like to show the vast amount of variety that can be utilized starting with lunch. There are so many different foods and meal choices but they are all in similar balance as you will learn. Again, just choose one option out of each category given or you can come up with your own creation. A turkey sandwich is a good example meal. Bread=carbohydrate, cheese=fat, turkey=protein, lettuce and tomato=color. You can start with the sandwich for convenience sake or mix and match. Below are example alternatives for each ingredient contained in the sandwich which can be used to create a whole new meal option.

Bread/Carbohydrate Alternates=

Whole grain cous cous

Whole grain pasta

Brown rice

Quinoa

Whole grain pita/wrap

Sweet potato

Whole grain crackers

Cheese/Fat alternates=

Olive oil and olive oil based dressings (e.g. vinaigrettes, pesto and other dressings)

Seeds (sunflower, sesame, flax)

Avocado

Whole butter

Mayonnaise (I prefer olive oil mayo)

A small quantity of nuts

Turkey-protein alternates=

Egg whites

Tilapia

Tuna

Boneless skinless chicken breast

Tofu

White (very low fat) ground turkey

Lean cuts of pork

0% yogurt

0% cottage cheese

0% milk

Protein and Fat Combo alternates= these foods count as both!

Salmon

Part skim mozzarella cheese

Peanut and almond butter

Red meats

Larger quantities of nuts

2% yogurt

2% cottage cheese

1% milk

Vegetarian Combinations- Legumes combined with seeds, nuts or grains.

Beans and rice, whole grain pasta, tortilla or toast

Lentils and wheat or rice

Hummus, pita and veggies

Peas and whole grain pasta or split pea soup with whole grain or seeded crackers

Note: Color options include every fruit and vegetable on planet earth, but try to keep fruits to a minimum at night and use them for their energy during the day. You should get at least eight servings of fruits and vegetables but only three of them should be from fruits. The serving should consist of 1 ½ cup of fruit or veggies but 1 cup *must be* a serving size for leafy greens. Focus on veggies for your color at night because they are always a great option. Try to use the more sugary vegetables like carrots, peas and corn sparingly in the evening.

Step 4: Choose your afternoon snack. It's getting later in the day now and in general people's schedules slow down a little at this time. You will still need carbohydrates, but it's time to start thinking about trimming them down. I use whole grain crackers as an example because people seem to like them. They're easy to pack and they contain a controlled amount of carbohydrates, low sugar and are a good fiber option but you can use anything comparable such as half piece of toast.

Different examples of good choices would be:

1.   1 Apple, 10 almonds and a few crackers or 1 apple and 15 almonds. Depending on your activity level, you may require the whole grain crackers to keep your glucose base up and stable. If your activity level is going to be mild or nonexistent then you may not need the crackers because the sugar and fiber in the apple along

with the fiber, fat and protein in the almonds may do the trick.

2.   Cheese/peanut butter/almond butter, fruit and a couple of crackers/1/2 whole wheat toast

3.   2% Yogurt with small amount of cereal, if any.

4.   2% Cottage cheese with or without a couple of crackers or   wheat germ.

5.   Hummus and veggies

6.   2 hard-boiled eggs and crudités (raw vegetables cut in bite size strips)

Step 5: Create a dinner. Go for zero carbs, or at least, very little carbs. Most of us don't do anything after dinner, and when mechanical activity slows so should carbohydrate intake. For this reason I usually strip pasta, rice, bread and potatoes etc. from dinner when I am designing programs in the beginning if it is right for the individual. Usually, people are used to having a mound of carbohydrates at night. This is, of course, due to the neglect of blood sugar levels earlier in the day and the cravings that are a result of those bad decisions. Choose your protein source first and assess it for its fat content and remember one fat source only. If it's salmon or red meat, your fat intake is covered, but if it's a white fish or chicken breast then you need to add fat to the meal. If you're dining out, stay away from choices with fatty sauces. Go lean and green, add another color and choose a sensible fat source. You can add fat to the pan to cook but for now, it is best to bake in water or pan fry in cooking spray and add olive oil (or other quality oils) to your meal after cooking it. Aside from the caloric accountability factor, room temperature oil is best for you.

As discussed earlier, unsaturated fats, like olive oil, have a tendency to break down molecularly when heated and cross bond when cooled making them less effective, prone to rancidity and harder to utilize in the body. You are shooting for 2 cups of veggies at dinner. Remember that you must get two different colors and alternate between raw and cooked.   Different colors are a necessity because we need a broad spectrum of earth chemical (phytochemicals) profiles.   You need to alternate from cooking to raw because cooking veggies breaks down fibrous content and causes loss of nutrients. You can eat raw all of the time, but you can't eat cooked all the time. Whether one night you do 1 cup cooked and 1 cup raw, or all cooked another night and all raw the following night or simply raw *all* the time. Whichever way works best for you is fine… you just want to do it. As you start getting closer to achieving your goals or if you tend to be more active, small amounts of carbs will be introduced to your meals. I have learned that in most home environments, the woman is far more active in the evening than the man.   Often times in program design, this needs to be considered but shouldn't be a concern.

6. The sixth meal and the late night snack

Due to the long duration between dinner and breakfast, your body enters a fasting state when asleep at night. To avoid catabolism or if you are going to be awake for more than three hours after dinner, you need to eat again.   Avoid substantial carbohydrates or anything with high fat content. Pure protein and veggie is what you should be going for at this time of the day. You require less energy at night, so why would you fill your body with high power fuels like carbs and fat? Keeping easy access, pre- portioned snacks available in the fridge is important. Personally, I like to have a few hard boiled eggs or a scoop of chocolate protein powder handy (use a shaker and just add cold water), but there are lots of other great options. Try some of these options: 3 oz., pre portioned (on Sunday) baggies of chicken or turkey breast ready to have alone or to dip with a little mustard and sliced veggies! Low fat cottage cheese and a low sugar/fat yogurt is great too because the kind of protein they contain has a timed release effect that promotes protection from catabolism deep into the night. Also, both yogurt and cottage cheese are very low in lactose because the lactose content is drastically reduced during fermentation for the lactose intolerant crowd. A palm size amount of edamame (soy beans) is also an option for women. Men should keep intake of flax seeds and soy to a minimum due to their estrogenic effects. You can choose one of these options and modify it to your liking or come up with something totally new. The important thing to remember is that you keep protein and low sugar veggies your focus.

10. Section Four: Preparation and Environmental Control

Victory favors the prepared!

Many of the people who first hear about how this program works as far as preparation and accountability say: "You just don't know how crazy my schedule is...my job, my kids, my social life, my school schedule, my, my, my." Allow me to let you in on a little secret...your schedule is not special. You are just like me and anyone else who is living a hectic life no matter how it varies. So, that is not an excuse, it's a "cop out". In fact, if you prioritize just a little bit of time towards preparation, you can turn your chaotic day into a day consisting of order, structure, ease and peace, but most importantly, you will be creating time. Well over ten thousand clients, and counting, have achieved complete success by following this very simple guideline of maintaining accountability for their intake. Even the clients, who don't do it perfectly, still see great change due to the awareness it created. But that will not be you! You need to go into this new lifestyle with a submissive attitude. Forfeit all control to the process just for a while until you become proficient and self-sufficient in all that you're trying to achieve for your body. Your body is a beautiful, majestic thing, in any condition, at any age! You should respect it as such. It is capable of incredible feats... you need only give it the right environment to blossom.

Preparation breeds adherence. If you put in work towards preparing structure for the following day, that effort will give you that certain feeling that you're building something that will not be easily torn down. That's what this section is all about, controlling your environment! Your environment is controlled in two ways: controlling your surrounding influences, and controlling and protecting your "internal" environment... your personal biochemistry. To control your internal environment, we have designed your perfect day, which you will be executing with precision, every day for two weeks.

Now you may ask, "What if I'm going out to dinner one night?" That's no problem... simply fall back on the five principles and do your best to control what outside chemicals enter your internal environment. Follow these pointers: 1) you know that you *must* stay away from Carbohydrates...that's non-negotiable. It's night time and there is no reason for you to light your fire. 2) You already know how many fats are allowed per meal, only one. Therefore, choose your protein and assess it for fat. If it has a significant fat source, don't add one. If it doesn't contain a significant source, get one, and consider what kind of fat it is and if it fits in your day. If you've already had a lot of fat, order the salmon instead of the steak. Now all you need is your two different colored veggies and you're all set. No matter where you are, your environment does not have power over you as long as you fall back on the five principles.

1. Eat within ½ hour of waking.

2. Make sure all meals during the day contain complex carbohydrate and at night cut them way down or out.

3. Eat every three hours.

4. Have only one fat per meal.

5. Plan and be accountable.

These five simple things will give you more control in what feels like uncontrollable environments. Over time, you will truly see the power of these simple principles as they catalyze change. When you find yourself unable to get hold of your committed foods you need for your perfect day of eating, always fall back on the principles. Most days you will find that you can stick to your perfect day, and just to reinforce adherence to the program, here are the steps to achieving control... *do not* deviate from any of them, even for a second.

1. Prepare and Pack Meals 2, 3 and 4 the Night Before

Even if you won't be going anywhere the following day, you still need to **pack *for* that day**. Do not pack your food in the morning! Go to bed tonight knowing that tomorrow is taken care of, no exceptions. Also, prepare your foods for Saturdays and Sundays the nights before. Be sure to pack your cooler bag containing your meals, food log (with your perfect day on page one), and a pen so that you isolate the nutrients required for your body for the following day. All that your body needs is in the bag! Touch nothing else.

Make Sunday your preparation day. Cook, cut, and portion (separate) your foods for the week on Sunday, e.g. containers of cut veggies, 3oz baggies of chicken for sandwiches, salads, late snacks, or fast dinners etc. Wednesday is another great preparation day for mid-week, if you can't or prefer not to prepare your whole week of food on Sundays.

2. Write Everything Down: Your Perception is Not Reality

By limiting your variety for the first two weeks, food tracking is made easier and creates accountability. Remember, you can't have variety and accountability in the beginning. Variety is the enemy of accountability. Once you get the hang of it and have seen some changes, you can begin to cycle in other food combinations using your newfound knowledge, and before you know it, you can eat whatever you want! That's the beauty of this education based system. In just a little time and with a little practice, you can eat what you want, feel how you want, look how you want, and get what you want! Now that's living. Track everything! No matter what happens. If you make a mistake and fall off for a day, you must write everything down to get back on track. Do not focus your energy towards being upset about the mistake. The only time you should feel like you're really slipping is if you don't log your intake. You will learn from it and make a better decision the next time you encounter the same situation. If fat loss stops and you can't figure out why, it's because you stopped writing it down. Start writing again and your fat loss will start again too. You may think you are doing everything right, but if you're not writing everything down, you are slipping. Your mental account of what is happening is frequently inaccurate, and when you start to write and review again you will see that in the record of your week. Don't let it get to that point and stay diligent.

3. The "Red Pen Head Check" and Weigh in.

After logging every item that passes your lips for the first week, it's time for the red pen acknowledgement of wrong and right doings. With a red pen or highlighter, carefully go through each day of your log and using the criteria of the five principles, circle and analyze the defects in your week e.g. salmon, avocado and veggies for dinner, circle the avocado and next to it write, "2 fats". This may sound silly but be sure to give yourself stars, check marks or smiley faces for the days that you execute perfectly. Collect as many as you can... count them and acknowledge them out loud! The closer to perfect you get, the faster the fat falls off, your energy increases, lean mass improves and the quicker you feel incredible. For every deviation from your plan, the results slow down. If you have a bad day, simply write it all down and hit the reset button. Say reset button out loud to audibly confirm your action! Do not waste energy on being negative. Instead, focus that energy towards pressuring the process and everything will go your way. The goal is to collect nothing but star's and smiley faces leaving nothing left to circle as you work toward perfection! Weigh in on the same day of the week that you grade your log, and *only* that day. I like Wednesdays for checking in because it allows you time to recover from weekend indulgences that you will have later during the final stage…maintenance.

4. Portions- No scale needed

The last thing you want to do is create a "medicinal" type of relationship with food. To maintain a healthy relationship with your food on an emotional, cultural, sociological and physiological level, you need to learn to trust your own judgment of quantity and quality. Leave these following items on your kitchen counter to reference for the first two weeks, then get rid of them and trust yourself!

1. Match box = 1oz

2. Deck of cards = 3oz

3. Measuring cup= 1 cup

5. Set the alarms

Set three alarms on your cell phone for meals 2, 3 and 4. Do not skip this step… it is of major importance even though right now, it might seem unnecessary. That's your pride getting in the way of your success. Hand over the controls and do it my way, and you will not be sorry. If you pack the next day's meals 2, 3, and 4 the night before and you put your food log and pen in the bag with the food, you can easily write every meal down as the day goes along. Also, set your alarms and you will not fail. Leave any of these details out of your daily routine at your own risk! Everything can be so easy if you follow the rules and are prepared. If you do not, you'll make everything harder on yourself and end up blaming it on everything other than your own lack of following directions.

Make sure that all of these steps are done before you go to bed and the next day will be a breeze. Wake up and eat your specified breakfast. Three hours later, when the alarm goes off, eat meal two and write it down; and so on… it's that simple. Execute and track your first perfect day, repeat and enjoy.

I can't begin to express the importance of these steps enough especially during the first twenty-one to thirty days. Do it. Don't worry if you're in a meeting and it goes long when the alarm goes off. As soon as you can, without putting too much pressure on any social engagement, get that food in you and if you have to eat early because of a bind, go for it. I would much rather you eat a little early than late. Don't sweat it if you have to eat early… simply eat three hours after **that** meal and everything is back on track. Don't worry if it's not exact, but definitely strive for perfection. Make it a game you're playing! Collect as many perfect days as possible and try to get the high score!

11. Section Five: Expanding Variety and Maintaining Your Results

After your first two weeks of preparing, eating and recording your perfect day, it's about time to start designing alternate meal choices that meet the criteria. You don't necessarily have to switch yet, but you do have to get in the habit of formulating proper macro nutrient ratios to match your lifestyle. Some people can't wait for the variety to begin so they rush in and change things early, while others tend to get too comfortable with the same foods and don't want to change. Both tendencies are bad. Take your time designing an alternative for each meal and transition as you are comfortable. Be methodical. Do not waver from the five principals and you will reach your goal. Remember, it's not the particular foods, it's the way you are pairing them. The strict accountability is not forever but the education is, so use the skill set you have acquired. When you do reach your goal, you will be able to "party", whatever that means to you, on the weekends and never have to worry about gaining back the weight or feeling guilty.

During the week, keep to the principles (which at this point are only four because you no longer write it down) and on the weekends you cut loose a little... eat what you want. Every Wednesday when you check your scale, you will have maintained your results. You will probably even lose a little more fat slowly over time and "tighten up" even further because indulging a little can stimulate your metabolism. This, of course, comes after you have earned a fast metabolism over time and achieved your initial goal. After creating new perfect days over and over again, it becomes second nature and you become a master of creating balanced, creative, delicious, and nutritious meals in any environment.

You have, at this point, acquired some well-earned freedom. The ability to eat what you want, look how you want, physically do what you want, and get what you want. This dramatically improves every single aspect of your life! When you reach your goal, you will find that you are capable of a lot more physically and you're in a whole new place mentally. If desired, set new goals and go after them, continue your education, investigate and grow or just relax into your new found abilities and enjoy the fact that your desperate pursuit of change is over and put that chapter of your life to bed. Either way, it's an incredibly empowering feeling to gain that kind of control and it completely enhances the experience of being a human being on planet earth.

In summary

No matter what your goal is, preparation and accountability are of the most important factors to focus on. If they are not in place, you're not on track. Whether you are trying to lose fat, improve performance, increase energy, gain muscle mass or just optimize your overall health in today's fast paced world, you must prepare to make balanced meals available at a second's notice. Furthermore, write your intake down to maintain an accountability and awareness of every unit of heat (calorie) that enters your body. For this reason, variety should be limited when initially starting a new regimen. You must be sick of hearing this, but it's *fundamental* to your journey...though the spice of life, variety is the enemy of accountability. The goal is to have absolute control. Accept nothing less! After two weeks of maintaining that control and seeing results, you will have started to adapt to the new regime and will be motivated by the change you see and feel. It is at this point, that it's safe to slowly integrate new foods. Next are a few things that will help you along the way. **Cook and separate portions on Sundays and pack your cooler**

bag the night before. Include your food log and pen and make sure you write down everything as it happens... not later as you remember it. Last, but not least, remember the **key** point of **preparation and accountability.** Set your cell phone's alarms for meal times. Most of us are extremely connected to our cell phones... every beep and buzz. We are going to use that to our advantage. **Prepare to succeed or plan to fail!**

12. SPECIAL POPULATIONS:

Stop blaming it on GENETIC PREDISPOSITION!

High Cholesterol:

It is true that genetic characteristics are passed down from generation to generation but you know what is also passed down? Bad habits and the latter are more likely the cause of your high cholesterol. Here is how it works: Your blood is comprised of red blood cells, white blood cells, platelets and plasma. Platelets have the important job of clotting together to stop bleeding as well as carrying growth factors that promote cell reproduction. The platelets are oval in shape and should easily tumble in transit through the blood stream. However, with high amounts of low density lipoproteins (LDL), plaque (made up of fat, calcium, cholesterol and cellular debris) begins to develop on the arterial walls, and the platelets begin to slide up against arterial walls and each other and get "stuck". Plaque causes the artery to become brittle (arthrosclerosis) and the plaque can begin to occlude(close up) the arteries promoting high blood pressure and an overall breakdown of the circulatory system which in turn negatively affects all functions in the body.

Even with genetic pre-disposition or elevated cholesterol levels there are tools at your disposal that will significantly reduce and/or eradicate high cholesterol. Here is a different way to look at it: cholesterol is a good thing, and is responsible for things such as cell membrane function, absorption of dietary fat, the synthesis of vitamin D and the synthesis of bile salts. In fact, up to two thirds of the cholesterol that enters the body every day comes from your own liver. Our bodies make a lot of cholesterol. When we consume large amounts of dietary cholesterol, the liver slows its production, but it can only down-regulate its production so much. The liver contributes to digestion through production of bile (made of bile salts, bile pigments and cholesterol). Bile assists the body's ability to absorb fat by emulsification (mixing fat with water). To keep up with digestion, bile has to be recycled, and during the recycling process, soluble fiber binds to bile salts causing them to be excreted. Since cholesterol is required to make new bile, more soluble fiber can lower your cholesterol. Pretty cool, huh?

Soluble fiber and mono unsaturated fats are the solution, along with all of the other principles in place of course! Apple and almonds anyone? More mono unsaturated fats are needed to change the LDL to HDL and support a "nonstick" environment and more soluble fiber to help lower overall cholesterol by removing bile salt and forcing the use of cholesterol to make more bile and keep the arteries clean! Over time, as the plaque is removed and further build up is avoided, the walls of the arteries can begin to go back to a soft, supple state. This combination solves the problem of high cholesterol. More than ten thousand people later and it still works every time! We will discuss how to apply this properly in further detail later in the program/design portion of the text.

High blood pressure: Hypertension

High blood pressure is virtually nonexistent in more remote and less developed parts of the world and in the elderly populations as well. Making lifestyle changes towards better nutritional choices and stress control creates a huge impact on high blood pressure, but make no mistake about it...stress is the lesser contributor of the two. Diets high in animal fat, high sodium intake and obesity are the main culprits. Smoking, caffeine intake and alcohol are also big factors. Heavy and consistent alcohol consumption is the biggest factor of the three.

High sodium intake seems to be more damaging when levels of potassium and magnesium are low. Lowering your sodium intake is a great step but you should also add more food choices that have high potassium, magnesium and calcium content (fruits and veggies). This is how it goes: high cholesterol=plaque buildup=occluded and less flexible arteries=high blood pressure. High cholesterol, high blood pressure and type 2 diabetes are usually all connected. You can fix this and live a drug-free life by implementing all you have learned through this program, using the tools I've given you, and by increasing your exercise. If you are going to increase your exercise regimen but suffer from high blood pressure, always consult your doctor first about your plan for increasing movement. Nice long walks are incredible and usually safe for anyone. They create movement in a positive direction towards just about any goal! Eating a raw clove of garlic daily has also been shown to make a considerable difference in lowering blood pressure, helping to keep platelets from sticking and reducing fat in the blood.

Diabetes

Type II diabetes is a cellular resistance to insulin which results in an inability to metabolize glucose. This causes excess glucose levels in the blood which is toxic and makes diabetes the number one cause of blindness, heart disease, and kidney failure and limb amputations. It also affects the body's ability to utilize oxygen which negatively affects all function. It is no joke! Yet surprisingly, some people treat it as such. I have seen it's horrors but it's easily managed if not cured by making sure that you stabilize your glucose base and get leaner. That's right, I said *cured*, and I have thousands of documented cases to prove it, so once again, don't pull the genetic card on me, it won't work. Instead, use the many tools available to you to rid yourself of this "bad decision" disease once and for all.

Diabetes is caused by factors such as bad nutrition, (obviously) obesity and stress.   But trust me; stress is the least of the three. The worst limiting factors keeping us from ridding this country of the plague that is Type II diabetes is a lack of knowledge. It would also be nice if, in general, medicine would focus more on educating individuals with what works, instead of only treating symptoms which doesn't work!

Diabetes accounts for $100 billion dollars in healthcare spending annually. That's big business, so you better take it upon yourself to take care of it and it's not that hard. If thousands of my clients have done it, so can you. In most cases, to cure a condition, do what should have been done to avoid getting it in the first place. That always equates to maintaining biochemical stability which you learned all about in the previous portions of this text. So, use the principals, respect the fact that you have a working pancreas and treat it kindly. Type I diabetes is the rough one. Type I diabetic's dream of only having Type II because they can't even produce the required insulin. A working pancreas would be a "dream come true" for them. If you have any concerns about any blood sugar imbalances, chances are, you are Type II because only 5-10% of all diabetics are Type I. In my very long career of working with Type II diabetics, never have the methods I use in this book, failed in stabilizing morning and evening blood sugar readings. These methods also lowered or completely removed medication dependency with Physicians approval. In addition, these methods lowered "A1C" well below 7, clearing all symptoms. Type I diabetes is more complex depending on the individual's situation but the same principals apply. If you are Type I diabetic or Type II insulin dependent, make sure to work closely with your doctor when making these changes and explain your rationale to your doctor. This will help your doctor make insulin recommendations that work in harmony with your nutritional intake.

What needs to happen now is that all of the previously learned principles need to be applied to your life, but twice daily monitoring of blood sugar readings *must* be taken and an ever present awareness of how you feel is mandatory. Along with setting in place the rest of what you've learned, there are special considerations for diabetics. You obviously have to eat carbohydrates that are unprocessed and high in fiber and stay away from anything "white" until you get things under control. There must be no sweets! It's not "treat time" but if you do eat them consume when active and keep portions considerably low. Fruits and vegetables have great fiber that will act like a net or a sponge to suspend water and food particles that allows for slower entry into the blood. Remember to never drink juice, always eat the fruit because it comes with fiber. As far as sugars go, fructose (fruit sugar) has the lowest insulin response but high unused quantities are converted to triglycerides, stored fat. They increase the rate of cataract formation, contributing to blindness. Your best bet with fruit is to use it for its metabolic stimulating benefits and when active during the day. Keep the portions under close control and avoid them at night.

There are a host of supplements that can help support and protect your body's systems from the damage caused by diabetes as well as some that are known to promote better insulin sensitivity. However, rather than getting lost in the endless world of supplements, I will just review a couple that could be added if cleared by your doctor. Please note that rarely, if ever, do I suggest the idea of supplements when working with clients. Just by balancing food intake within the first two weeks, blood sugar levels are stable and all symptoms are reduced dramatically or eradicated altogether. So, what I'm saying is, most likely you don't even need them, but in severe cases these are a couple that I speak about with my clients and have clients ask their doctor about adding to their nutritional regime.

I'm going to focus on supplements that help improve how well your cells uptake glucose or your glucose tolerance level (GTL). Biotin, a B vitamin, works with insulin to improve the utilization of glucose and protect from neuropathy as well as helping hair, skin and nails. Vitamin C has been shown to reduce the need for insulin and help maintain eye health, and help with cataracts in diabetics. Even small deficiencies of chromium, magnesium and potassium can negatively affect the body's ability to use glucose. Other than that, essential fatty acids have been shown to decrease insulin resistance and amino acids supply the raw materials to manufacture insulin as they do for so many things. Insulin is actually a hormone that is made of 51 amino acids. I never get more in depth with supplementation than that because frankly, it probably isn't necessary.

One thing that *is* necessary is exercise. It mobilizes body fat for use as fuel and assists with GTL. Indeed, higher intensity use of your muscles causes the uptake of glucose for fuel without using insulin. Regular exercise is something that is very important to focus on. You don't have to get crazy with it, just be consistent and progress comfortably. Long walks are an unbelievable way to sizzle off fat and help with glucose use. A nice walk after dinner is a great habit to get into. We might take away carbohydrates almost completely at dinner for someone who is apparently healthy and eager to get aggressive towards their goals. I have found that with diabetics, making sure you have a little bit of high quality carbohydrate at dinner is a good idea until everything is under control. Excessive protein can hurt the kidneys and excessive fat is avoided because diabetics often have pancreatic enzyme deficiency which makes it hard to metabolize fat. So, because we can't increase fat and protein too much at dinner, we need that little bit of carbohydrates to balance everything out calorie wise.

As you can see it all comes down to balance, not just for diabetics, but for everyone. Let's face it... diabetes is a big part of a package deal with high cholesterol and high blood pressure.

It's not one condition but lately, it is treated as such. If you have one, you're probably doing things that are setting you up to having all three, and if you don't have anything wrong with you at all, these are still the same principles that you need to focus on to keep it that way and improve performance.

13. Beware of the Last Ten

If you have a fat loss goal ranging between 0 and 20 lbs., you need not worry about this section so much. Just follow the rules and you'll be there in no time. For the individuals that have a longer journey, beware of the last ten pounds. You will reach a point where you understand this so well that you can stop worrying about accountability as much. You may even reach a point where you can stop writing it down and still continue to make progress towards your goals. There is nothing wrong with that, in fact, you've earned it! But, there are three situations which demand that you go back to the kind of perfect accountability you started with:

1. When you hit within ten pounds of your final goal weight.

2. If during your progress the scale ever goes backwards.

3. Or, if after achieving your goal and while maintaining, you start to creep too close to your unacceptable number...a number you choose to never let yourself go beyond again unless it is your goal to do so.

Many of my clients get within ten pounds of complete success and get too comfortable. They have achieved a great level of education and an ability to control their environment and they get a little too comfortable and dare I say, cocky. They start to make every excuse in the book and blame everything but themselves for their lack of progress. The truth is that 100% of the time it comes down to the person being too stubborn to go back to the principles that ensured success from the beginning. You're never too smart to stop using the proven methods of preparation and tracking you employed in the beginning. Take away variety for two weeks, pack the night before, write down everything, and set the alarms on your phone or the last ten pounds will probably be rough.

Others have the opposite problem. They get to the last ten pounds and are not mentally prepared to stop. Sometimes this is due to self-image issues or stress, etc. You need to be sure to remember that the root idea behind all of this is to protect and care for your body, so stay within the guidelines. Aesthetics can be a mirage at first and sometimes it takes a while to get adjusted to the new you. If flabby skin troubles you after shedding some fat, remember that your skin contains a protein called elastin that will help to tighten loose skin over 6-9 months. Give it time to do its job. It is true that as we age levels of elastin lowers, but no matter the age, do not get any kind of surgery for at least nine months after losing weight. People tend to lose weight in sections. This of course can vary due to genetic differences, but it usually starts with the face, neck and shoulders.

After this initial phase, you begin to lose from the midsection, limbs and hips and finally the last to go is the lower abdomen. However, some people often worry that they will continue to lose in the face and become sick looking and out of proportion, and subsequently, they stray when they see this or if somebody, who is usually "over fat" themselves, makes a statement regarding your weight loss and appearance.

It never ceases to amaze me how often the people who are most critical of this program are the ones who end up in my office sitting across from me because of their doctor's recommendation. They demand that they create balance and change under the threat of death. There are a lot of psychological factors that try to take hold and many tricks your mind will try to play. Pay them no attention and trust the numbers. Keep going until you get within recommended weight and body fat levels. There will be plenty of play between "hard body" and a little curvier.

The guidelines are there so you always know your target and can trust it regardless of the head games. When you allow a little time to pass, it will really become clear just how incredible you look and feel about the **new you**. Remember, going too low in body fat and weight has ugly health consequences, especially in women. Hair, skin and nails are negatively affected as well as diminished hormone levels, weakened immune function, overall physiological imbalance, loss of sleep and dark circles under the eyes, naming a few. When you reach your goals you will have to remember that you can and should have some fun and enjoy yourself a little. Keep in mind that indulging on the weekend at this point can actually stimulate your metabolism.

You will never go backwards! You will be far too educated and in control. Incidentally, in 2002, I lost one hundred pounds. I applied the principles, put in the effort and experienced the dramatic changes personally and so will you! State your goals out loud! Tell everyone! Define this moment with a powerful voice! Write it down in **LARGE** letters and post it on your fridge! Pressure this process! Take what's yours! **Enjoy your results!**

Example 1

Meal 1 **Breakfast** Hungometer # _____	Time: 6:00AM Cal : 225	1 Cup Cereal ½ Cup 1% Milk ½ Banana	- 120 - 50 - 55
Meal 2 **Snack 1** Hungometer # _____	Time: 9:00 AM Cal : 220	0% Greek Yogurt ¼ Cup Cereal 1 Tbsp Sliced Almonds	- 140 - 30 - 50
Meal 3 **Lunch** Hungometer # _____	Time: 12:00PM Cal : 320	2 Slices Whole Grain Bread 3 Oz Turkey 1 Slice Low Fat Cheese Veggies	- 140 - 100 - 60 - 20
Meal 4 **Snack 2** Hungometer # _____	Time: 3:00PM Cal : 180	15 Almonds Apple	- 100 - 80
Meal 5 **Dinner** Hungometer # _____	Time: 6:00PM Cal : 280	4 Oz Salmon 2 Cups Cooked Veggies	- 200 - 80
Meal 6 **Late protein** **Snack**	Time: 9:00 PM Cal : 75	Hard Boiled egg	- 75
Total Calories _____	Supplements: Oz water :		

No Caloric Limit – 1,200 to ∞

Example 2

Meal 1 **Breakfast** Hungometer # _____	Time: 7:00 AM Cal : 215	1 Whole Wheat Wrap 3 Egg Whites 1 Tbsp Shredded Cheese 1/3 Cup Peppers & Onion	- 110 - 60 - 30 - 15
Meal 2 **Snack 1** Hungometer # _____	Time: 10:00 AM Cal : 180	Bar of your choice (must contain whole grain)	- 180
Meal 3 **Lunch** Hungometer # _____	Time: 1:00 PM Cal : 340	1 Pita (whole Grain) 4 oz Grilled Chicken 1 Tbsp Olive Oil Mayo Veggies	- 110 - 160 - 50 - 20
Meal 4 **Snack 2** Hungometer # _____	Time: 4:00 PM Cal : 220	1/3 Cup Hummus 3/4 Cup Carrots 3 Whole Grain Crackers	- 160 - 40 - 20
Meal 5 **Dinner** Hungometer # _____	Time: 7:00 PM Cal : 290	4 oz Filet Mignon 2 Cups Cooked Veggies	- 210 - 80
Meal 6 **Late protein** **Snack**	Time: 10:00 PM Cal : 100	1 Scoop Protein Powder (with Cold Water)	- 100
Total Calories _____	Supplements: Oz water :		

No Caloric Limit – 1,200 to ∞

Example 3

Meal 1 **Breakfast** Hungometer # _____	Time: 8:00 AM Cal : 230	½ Cup Cooked Oats 1 Tbsp Peanut Butter ¼ Cup 0% Milk ⅓ Blue Berries	- 75 - 100 - 25 - 30
Meal 2 **Snack 1** Hungometer # _____	Time: 11:00 AM Cal : 220	¾ Cup Low Fat Cottage Cheese ½ Cup Pineapple 5 Whole Grain Crackers	- 150 - 40 - 30
Meal 3 **Lunch** Hungometer # _____	Time: 2:00 PM Cal : 315	½ Cup Whole Grain Pasta 3 oz Chopped Grilled Chicken ⅓ Cup Mushrooms & Onion 2 tsp Pesto	- 100 - 120 - 15 - 80
Meal 4 **Snack 2** Hungometer # _____	Time: 5:00 PM Cal : 225	2 Low Fat Cheese Sticks ¾ Cup Grapes 10 Whole Grain Pretzels	- 120 - 75 - 30
Meal 5 **Dinner** Hungometer # _____	Time: 8:00 PM Cal : 330	4 oz Grilled Chicken 2 tsp Olive Oil 2 Tbsp Balsamic Vinegar 2 Cups Fresh Veggies	- 160 - 80 - 30 - 60
Meal 6 **Late protein** **Snack**	Time: 11:00 PM Cal :	½ Cup Shelled Edamame	- 100
Total Calories _____	Supplements: Oz water :		

No Caloric Limit – 1,200 to ∞

Example 4

Date: _____

Meal 1 **Breakfast** Hungometer # _____	Time: 9:00 AM Cal : 210	1 Whole Wheat English Muffin-100 1 Whole Egg - 75 1 Egg White - 20 1 Slice Tomato - 15
Meal 2 **Snack 1** Hungometer # _____	Time: 12:00 PM Cal : 195	1 Large Whole Grain Cracker - 40 1 Tbsp Almond Butter -100 ½ Banana - 55
Meal 3 **Lunch** Hungometer # _____	Time: 3:00 PM Cal : 270	½ Cup Brown Rice - 100 ⅓ Cup Black Beans - 80 ½ Cup Pico de Gallo - 30 1 Tbsp Shredded Cheese - 30 1 Tbsp Non-fat Sour Cream -30
Meal 4 **Snack 2** Hungometer # _____	Time: 6:00 PM Cal : 210	1 Scoop Protein Powder - 100 (with Cold Water) 10 Almonds (Raw) - 80 ½ Cup Strawberries - 30
Meal 5 **Dinner** Hungometer # _____	Time: 9:00 PM Cal : 275	6 oz Tilapia -165 1 Tbsp Olive Oil Mayo - 50 2 Cups Veggies - 60
Meal 6 **Late protein** **Snack**	Time: 12:00 AM Cal :	3 oz Chicken Breast Strips -120 (Grilled)
Total Calories _____	Supplements: Oz water :	

No Caloric Limit – 1,200 to ∞

Design Your Perfect Day Here

Nutrition Log:

Date: _____

Meal 1 Breakfast hungometer# _____	Time:_____ Cal:_____
Meal 2 Snack 1 hungometer# _____	Time:_____ Cal:_____
Meal 3 Lunch hungometer# _____	Time:_____ Cal:_____
Meal 4 Snack 2 hungometer# _____	Time:_____ Cal:_____
Meal 5 Dinner hungometer# _____	Time:_____ Cal:_____
Meal 6 late protein Snack hungometer# _____	Time:_____ Cal:_____
Total Calories _____	Supplements: Oz water:

NO CALORIC LIMIT - 1200 to ∞

Nutrition Log:

Date: _____

Meal 1 Breakfast hungometer# _____	Time:_____ Cal:_____
Meal 2 Snack 1 hungometer# _____	Time:_____ Cal:_____
Meal 3 Lunch hungometer# _____	Time:_____ Cal:_____
Meal 4 Snack 2 hungometer# _____	Time:_____ Cal:_____
Meal 5 Dinner hungometer# _____	Time:_____ Cal:_____
Meal 6 late protein Snack hungometer# _____	Time:_____ Cal:_____
Total Calories _____	Supplements: Oz water:

NO CALORIC LIMIT - 1200 to ∞

Nutrition Log:

Date: _____

Meal 1 Breakfast hungometer# _____	Time:_____ Cal:_____
Meal 2 Snack 1 hungometer# _____	Time:_____ Cal:_____
Meal 3 Lunch hungometer# _____	Time:_____ Cal:_____
Meal 4 Snack 2 hungometer# _____	Time:_____ Cal:_____
Meal 5 Dinner hungometer# _____	Time:_____ Cal:_____
Meal 6 late protein Snack hungometer# _____	Time:_____ Cal:_____
Total Calories _____	Supplements: Oz water:

NO CALORIC LIMIT - 1200 to ∞

Nutrition Log:

Date: _____

Meal 1 Breakfast hungometer# _____	Time:_____ Cal:_____
Meal 2 Snack 1 hungometer# _____	Time:_____ Cal:_____
Meal 3 Lunch hungometer# _____	Time:_____ Cal:_____
Meal 4 Snack 2 hungometer# _____	Time:_____ Cal:_____
Meal 5 Dinner hungometer# _____	Time:_____ Cal:_____
Meal 6 late protein Snack hungometer# _____	Time:_____ Cal:_____
Total Calories _____	Supplements: Oz water:

NO CALORIC LIMIT - 1200 to ∞

Nutrition Log:

Date: _____

Meal 1 Breakfast hungometer# _____	Time:_____ Cal:_____
Meal 2 Snack 1 hungometer# _____	Time:_____ Cal:_____
Meal 3 Lunch hungometer# _____	Time:_____ Cal:_____
Meal 4 Snack 2 hungometer# _____	Time:_____ Cal:_____
Meal 5 Dinner hungometer# _____	Time:_____ Cal:_____
Meal 6 late protein Snack hungometer# _____	Time:_____ Cal:_____
Total Calories _____	Supplements: Oz water:

NO CALORIC LIMIT - 1200 to ∞

Nutrition Log:

Date: _____

Meal 1 Breakfast hungometer# _____	Time:_____ Cal:_____
Meal 2 Snack 1 hungometer# _____	Time:_____ Cal:_____
Meal 3 Lunch hungometer# _____	Time:_____ Cal:_____
Meal 4 Snack 2 hungometer# _____	Time:_____ Cal:_____
Meal 5 Dinner hungometer# _____	Time:_____ Cal:_____
Meal 6 late protein Snack hungometer# _____	Time:_____ Cal:_____
Total Calories _____	Supplements: Oz water:

NO CALORIC LIMIT - 1200 to ∞

Nutrition Log:

Date: _____

Meal 1 Breakfast hungometer# _____	Time:_____ Cal:_____
Meal 2 Snack 1 hungometer# _____	Time:_____ Cal:_____
Meal 3 Lunch hungometer# _____	Time:_____ Cal:_____
Meal 4 Snack 2 hungometer# _____	Time:_____ Cal:_____
Meal 5 Dinner hungometer# _____	Time:_____ Cal:_____
Meal 6 late protein Snack hungometer# _____	Time:_____ Cal:_____
Total Calories _____	Supplements: Oz water:

NO CALORIC LIMIT - 1200 to ∞

Nutrition Log:

Date: _____

Meal 1 Breakfast hungometer# _____	Time:_____ Cal:_____
Meal 2 Snack 1 hungometer# _____	Time:_____ Cal:_____
Meal 3 Lunch hungometer# _____	Time:_____ Cal:_____
Meal 4 Snack 2 hungometer# _____	Time:_____ Cal:_____
Meal 5 Dinner hungometer# _____	Time:_____ Cal:_____
Meal 6 late protein Snack hungometer# _____	Time:_____ Cal:_____
Total Calories _____	Supplements: Oz water:

NO CALORIC LIMIT - 1200 to ∞

Nutrition Log:

Date: _____

Meal 1 Breakfast hungometer# _____	Time:_____ Cal:_____
Meal 2 Snack 1 hungometer# _____	Time:_____ Cal:_____
Meal 3 Lunch hungometer# _____	Time:_____ Cal:_____
Meal 4 Snack 2 hungometer# _____	Time:_____ Cal:_____
Meal 5 Dinner hungometer# _____	Time:_____ Cal:_____
Meal 6 late protein Snack hungometer# _____	Time:_____ Cal:_____
Total Calories _____	Supplements: Oz water:

NO CALORIC LIMIT - 1200 to ∞

Nutrition Log:

Date: _____

Meal 1 Breakfast hungometer# _____	Time:_____ Cal:_____
Meal 2 Snack 1 hungometer# _____	Time:_____ Cal:_____
Meal 3 Lunch hungometer# _____	Time:_____ Cal:_____
Meal 4 Snack 2 hungometer# _____	Time:_____ Cal:_____
Meal 5 Dinner hungometer# _____	Time:_____ Cal:_____
Meal 6 late protein Snack hungometer# _____	Time:_____ Cal:_____
Total Calories _____	Supplements: Oz water:

NO CALORIC LIMIT - 1200 to ∞

Nutrition Log:

Date: _____

Meal 1 Breakfast hungometer# _____	Time:_____ Cal:_____
Meal 2 Snack 1 hungometer# _____	Time:_____ Cal:_____
Meal 3 Lunch hungometer# _____	Time:_____ Cal:_____
Meal 4 Snack 2 hungometer# _____	Time:_____ Cal:_____
Meal 5 Dinner hungometer# _____	Time:_____ Cal:_____
Meal 6 late protein Snack hungometer# _____	Time:_____ Cal:_____
Total Calories _____	Supplements: Oz water:

NO CALORIC LIMIT - 1200 to ∞

Nutrition Log:

Date: _____

Meal 1 Breakfast hungometer# _____	Time:_____ Cal:_____
Meal 2 Snack 1 hungometer# _____	Time:_____ Cal:_____
Meal 3 Lunch hungometer# _____	Time:_____ Cal:_____
Meal 4 Snack 2 hungometer# _____	Time:_____ Cal:_____
Meal 5 Dinner hungometer# _____	Time:_____ Cal:_____
Meal 6 late protein Snack hungometer# _____	Time:_____ Cal:_____
Total Calories _____	Supplements: Oz water:

NO CALORIC LIMIT - 1200 to ∞

Nutrition Log:

Date: _____

Meal 1 Breakfast hungometer# _____	Time:_____ Cal:_____
Meal 2 Snack 1 hungometer# _____	Time:_____ Cal:_____
Meal 3 Lunch hungometer# _____	Time:_____ Cal:_____
Meal 4 Snack 2 hungometer# _____	Time:_____ Cal:_____
Meal 5 Dinner hungometer# _____	Time:_____ Cal:_____
Meal 6 late protein Snack hungometer# _____	Time:_____ Cal:_____
Total Calories _____	Supplements: Oz water:

NO CALORIC LIMIT - 1200 to ∞

Nutrition Log:

Date: _____

Meal 1 Breakfast hungometer# _____	Time:_____ Cal:_____
Meal 2 Snack 1 hungometer# _____	Time:_____ Cal:_____
Meal 3 Lunch hungometer# _____	Time:_____ Cal:_____
Meal 4 Snack 2 hungometer# _____	Time:_____ Cal:_____
Meal 5 Dinner hungometer# _____	Time:_____ Cal:_____
Meal 6 late protein Snack hungometer# _____	Time:_____ Cal:_____
Total Calories _____	Supplements: Oz water:

NO CALORIC LIMIT - 1200 to ∞

Nutrition Log:

Date: _____

Meal 1 Breakfast hungometer# _____	Time:_____ Cal:_____
Meal 2 Snack 1 hungometer# _____	Time:_____ Cal:_____
Meal 3 Lunch hungometer# _____	Time:_____ Cal:_____
Meal 4 Snack 2 hungometer# _____	Time:_____ Cal:_____
Meal 5 Dinner hungometer# _____	Time:_____ Cal:_____
Meal 6 late protein Snack hungometer# _____	Time:_____ Cal:_____
Total Calories _____	Supplements: Oz water:

NO CALORIC LIMIT - 1200 to ∞

Nutrition Log:

Date: _____

Meal 1 Breakfast hungometer# _____	Time:_____ Cal:_____
Meal 2 Snack 1 hungometer# _____	Time:_____ Cal:_____
Meal 3 Lunch hungometer# _____	Time:_____ Cal:_____
Meal 4 Snack 2 hungometer# _____	Time:_____ Cal:_____
Meal 5 Dinner hungometer# _____	Time:_____ Cal:_____
Meal 6 late protein Snack hungometer# _____	Time:_____ Cal:_____
Total Calories _____	Supplements: Oz water:

NO CALORIC LIMIT - 1200 to ∞

Nutrition Log:

Date: _____

Meal 1 Breakfast hungometer# _____	Time:_____ Cal:_____
Meal 2 Snack 1 hungometer# _____	Time:_____ Cal._____
Meal 3 Lunch hungometer# _____	Time:_____ Cal:_____
Meal 4 Snack 2 hungometer# _____	Time:_____ Cal:_____
Meal 5 Dinner hungometer# _____	Time:_____ Cal:_____
Meal 6 late protein Snack hungometer# _____	Time:_____ Cal:_____
Total Calories _____	Supplements: Oz water:

NO CALORIC LIMIT - 1200 to ∞

Nutrition Log:

Date: _____

Meal 1 Breakfast hungometer# _____	Time:_____ Cal:_____
Meal 2 Snack 1 hungometer# _____	Time:_____ Cal:_____
Meal 3 Lunch hungometer# _____	Time:_____ Cal:_____
Meal 4 Snack 2 hungometer# _____	Time:_____ Cal:_____
Meal 5 Dinner hungometer# _____	Time:_____ Cal:_____
Meal 6 late protein Snack hungometer# _____	Time:_____ Cal:_____
Total Calories _____	Supplements: Oz water:

NO CALORIC LIMIT - 1200 to ∞

Nutrition Log:

Date: _____ __

Meal 1 Breakfast hungometer# _____	Time:_____ Cal:_____
Meal 2 Snack 1 hungometer# _____	Time:_____ Cal:_____
Meal 3 Lunch hungometer# _____	Time:_____ Cal:_____
Meal 4 Snack 2 hungometer# _____	Time:_____ Cal:_____
Meal 5 Dinner hungometer# _____	Time:_____ Cal:_____
Meal 6 late protein Snack hungometer# _____	Time:_____ Cal:_____
Total Calories _____	Supplements: Oz water:

NO CALORIC LIMIT - 1200 to ∞

Nutrition Log:

Date: _____

Meal 1 Breakfast hungometer# _____	Time:_____ Cal:_____
Meal 2 Snack 1 hungometer# _____	Time:_____ Cal:_____
Meal 3 Lunch hungometer# _____	Time:_____ Cal:_____
Meal 4 Snack 2 hungometer# _____	Time:_____ Cal:_____
Meal 5 Dinner hungometer# _____	Time:_____ Cal:_____
Meal 6 late protein Snack hungometer# _____	Time:_____ Cal:_____
Total Calories _____	Supplements: Oz water:

NO CALORIC LIMIT - 1200 to ∞

Nutrition Log:

Date: _____

Meal 1 Breakfast hungometer# _____	Time:_____ Cal:_____
Meal 2 Snack 1 hungometer# _____	Time:_____ Cal:_____
Meal 3 Lunch hungometer# _____	Time:_____ Cal:_____
Meal 4 Snack 2 hungometer# _____	Time:_____ Cal:_____
Meal 5 Dinner hungometer# _____	Time:_____ Cal:_____
Meal 6 late protein Snack hungometer# _____	Time:_____ Cal:_____
Total Calories _____	Supplements: Oz water:

NO CALORIC LIMIT - 1200 to ∞

Nutrition Log:

Date: _____

Meal 1 Breakfast hungometer# _____	Time:_____ Cal:_____
Meal 2 Snack 1 hungometer# _____	Time:_____ Cal:_____
Meal 3 Lunch hungometer# _____	Time:_____ Cal:_____
Meal 4 Snack 2 hungometer# _____	Time:_____ Cal:_____
Meal 5 Dinner hungometer# _____	Time:_____ Cal:_____
Meal 6 late protein Snack hungometer# _____	Time:_____ Cal:_____
Total Calories _____	Supplements: Oz water:

NO CALORIC LIMIT - 1200 to ∞

Nutrition Log:

Date: _____

Meal 1 Breakfast hungometer# _____	Time:_____ Cal:_____
Meal 2 Snack 1 hungometer# _____	Time:_____ Cal:_____
Meal 3 Lunch hungometer# _____	Time:_____ Cal:_____
Meal 4 Snack 2 hungometer# _____	Time:_____ Cal:_____
Meal 5 Dinner hungometer# _____	Time:_____ Cal:_____
Meal 6 late protein Snack hungometer# _____	Time:_____ Cal:_____
Total Calories _____	Supplements: Oz water:

NO CALORIC LIMIT - 1200 to ∞

Nutrition Log:

Date: _____

Meal 1 Breakfast hungometer# _____	Time:_____ Cal:_____
Meal 2 Snack 1 hungometer# _____	Time:_____ Cal:_____
Meal 3 Lunch hungometer# _____	Time:_____ Cal:_____
Meal 4 Snack 2 hungometer# _____	Time:_____ Cal:_____
Meal 5 Dinner hungometer# _____	Time:_____ Cal:_____
Meal 6 late protein Snack hungometer# _____	Time:_____ Cal:_____
Total Calories _____	Supplements: Oz water:

NO CALORIC LIMIT - 1200 to ∞

Nutrition Log:

Date: _____

Meal 1 Breakfast hungometer# _____	Time:_____ Cal:_____
Meal 2 Snack 1 hungometer# _____	Time:_____ Cal:_____
Meal 3 Lunch hungometer# _____	Time:_____ Cal:_____
Meal 4 Snack 2 hungometer# _____	Time:_____ Cal:_____
Meal 5 Dinner hungometer# _____	Time:_____ Cal:_____
Meal 6 late protein Snack hungometer# _____	Time:_____ Cal:_____
Total Calories _____ __	Supplements: Oz water:

NO CALORIC LIMIT - 1200 to ∞

Nutrition Log:

Date: _____

Meal 1 Breakfast hungometer# _____	Time:_____ Cal:_____
Meal 2 Snack 1 hungometer# _____	Time:_____ Cal:_____
Meal 3 Lunch hungometer# _____	Time:_____ Cal:_____
Meal 4 Snack 2 hungometer# _____	Time:_____ Cal:_____
Meal 5 Dinner hungometer# _____	Time:_____ Cal:_____
Meal 6 late protein Snack hungometer# _____	Time:_____ Cal:_____
Total Calories _____	Supplements: Oz water:

NO CALORIC LIMIT - 1200 to ∞

Nutrition Log:

Date: _____

Meal 1 Breakfast hungometer# _____	Time:_____ Cal._____
Meal 2 Snack 1 hungometer# _____	Time:_____ Cal: _____
Meal 3 Lunch hungometer# _____	Time:_____ Cal:_____
Meal 4 Snack 2 hungometer# _____	Time:_____ Cal:_____
Meal 5 Dinner hungometer# _____	Time:_____ Cal:_____
Meal 6 late protein Snack hungometer# _____	Time:_____ Cal:_____
Total Calories _____	Supplements: Oz water:

NO CALORIC LIMIT - 1200 to ∞

Nutrition Log:

Date: _____

Meal 1 Breakfast hungometer# _____	Time:_____ Cal:_____
Meal 2 Snack 1 hungometer# _____	Time:_____ Cal:_____
Meal 3 Lunch hungometer# _____	Time:_____ Cal:_____
Meal 4 Snack 2 hungometer# _____	Time:_____ Cal:_____
Meal 5 Dinner hungometer# _____	Time:_____ Cal:_____
Meal 6 late protein Snack hungometer# _____	Time:_____ Cal:_____
Total Calories _____	Supplements: Oz water:

NO CALORIC LIMIT - 1200 to ∞

Nutrition Log:

Date: _____

Meal 1 Breakfast hungometer# _____	Time:_____ Cal:_____
Meal 2 Snack 1 hungometer# _____	Time:_____ Cal:_____
Meal 3 Lunch hungometer# _____	Time:_____ Cal:_____
Meal 4 Snack 2 hungometer# _____	Time:_____ Cal:_____
Meal 5 Dinner hungometer# _____	Time:_____ Cal:_____
Meal 6 late protein Snack hungometer# _____	Time:_____ Cal:_____
Total Calories _____	Supplements: Oz water:

NO CALORIC LIMIT - 1200 to ∞

My1PerfectDay.com

23910026R00065

Made in the USA
Middletown, DE
07 September 2015